Brock / Springer Series in Contemporary Bioscience

A Researcher's Guide to
Scientific and Medical Illustrations

Brock/Springer Series in Contemporary Bioscience

Series Editor: Thomas D. Brock
University of Wisconsin–Madison

Mary Helen Briscoe

A Researcher's Guide to Scientific and Medical Illustrations

With 172 Figures

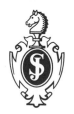

Springer-Verlag
New York Berlin Heidelberg
London Paris Tokyo Hong Kong

Mary Helen Briscoe
Medical Illustrator
Cardiovascular Research Institute
University of California, San Francisco
San Francisco, CA 94143, USA

Library of Congress Cataloging-in-Publication Data
Briscoe, Mary Helen.
  A researcher's guide to scientific and medical illustrations /
Mary Helen Briscoe.
    p. cm. — (Brock/Springer series in contemporary bioscience)
  Includes biographical references.
  ISBN 0-387-97199-8
1. Medical illustration. 2. Scientific illustration. I. Title.
II. Series.
  [DNLM: 1. Medical illustration. WZ 348 B859r]
R836.B73 1990
610′.22′2—dc20
DNLM/DLC   89-26214

Printed on acid-free paper.

Editorial supervision by Science Tech Publishers, Madison, Wisconsin.
Printed in the United States of America.

10 9 8 7 6 5 4 3 2 1

ISBN 0-387-97199-8 Springer-Verlag New York Berlin Heidelberg
ISBN 3-540-97199-8 Springer-Verlag Berlin Heidelberg New York

In memory of Julius H. Comroe, Jr.
without whom I would not have started,
and in gratitude to Wayne
without whom I would not have finished.

ACKNOWLEDGMENTS

For the many years' opportunity to practice and learn my profession, I am indebted to the Cardiovascular Research Institute (CVRI) and its director, Dr. Richard J. Havel. Many members of CVRI have been particularly helpful with their time, advice, and loan of books and figures. I am especially grateful to Dr. Norman Staub and students and faculty of his classes in The Art of Lecturing, Dr. Leonard Peller, Dr. Richard Bland, Dr. Donald MacDonald, Mr. Paul Graf, Ms. Rolinda Wang, Dr. Jen Tsi Yang, Dr. Wendy Wu, and to all who have given permission to use figures for this book.

Ms. Ilse Saurwald of the Department of Growth and Development took time to describe photographic processes and to develop and print some of the photographs. Dr. Geri Chen and Mr. David Hardman patiently demonstrated and explained the process of making, photographing, and printing gels.

For his expertise in explaining sequences and maps I am indebted to Dr. Hugo Martinez of the Department of Biochemistry and Biophysics of the University of California, San Francisco. Ms. Jori Mandelman, Dr. Martinez' assistant, generated most of the figures for the sequence and mapping sections and was also helpful with her explanations. The software developed by Dr. Martinez is remarkable for its wealth of detailed information and analytical capabilities. Its output is a basis for further hypotheses and experimentation.

Ms. Leslie Taylor of the Department of Pharmacy of the University of California, San Francisco, generously donated her time to explain and show molecular models generated in the computer graphics laboratory. Ms. Julie Newdoll, artist for the Department of Biochemistry and Biophysics of the University of California, San Francisco, was also helpful in explaining and demonstrating molecular models.

The advice, both scientific and literary, of Dr. Wayne Lanier has been invaluable, as has been the contribution of Mrs. Lilly Urbach in her perspicacious proof-reading.

I feel fortunate in having access to the resources of the University of California, San Francisco. The work being done here, the technical facilities, and the visiting scientists and lecturers have been a stimulus to continuing learning and teaching.

M.H.B.

CONTENTS

1

INTRODUCTION

In this age of communication and in this age of increasingly complex scientific research, effective communication is vital. Yet, good communication is difficult and rare, and poor communication hampers the development of the scientific enterprise. The reader or listener may become frustrated or exhausted at poorly presented information and lose interest. Examples abound of poorly presented papers. In fact, poor communication is becoming traditional at a time when understanding of science is crucial.

What Is Communication?

Communication is the giving of information to another, a sharing of intangibles.

To communicate is to be sociable and generous. It is a gracious and civilized act.

More pertinent to this book, communication is an essential factor in the development of science as a shared body of verified knowledge. Scientists, from the first, **openly** communicated their discoveries, thus distinguishing their work from that of astrologers, alchemists, and wizards.

Communication is a basic human function and, as such, is as necessary for survival now as it always has been. It is essential to the survival of science.

Communication requires participation and exchange: one giving, the other receiving. It is fluid and dynamic and should be rewarding and pleasurable to all concerned.

However, to the scientist who has done the work, the ideas are so familiar and clear that the necessity of making these ideas clear to others may not be obvious. Bald statements of fact may not be understood. Ways to organize, simplify, and emphasize facts are essential for clear communication.

An Intention to Communicate

In science, accuracy is vital. So also is a genuine intent to inform. Too often a stated intent to inform is belied by the other messages that communicate all too clearly, such as:

- Nobody is going to understand.
- See how much I know.
- I am too busy with important work to take pains with this.
- It is up to you to figure this out.

It is essential that the message be as accurate as the calculations. The scientist must make a commitment to inform. You must be interested in your own information if you want anyone else to find it interesting. Concentrate on finding ways to make your information clear and interesting to others.

Visual Communication

Communication is often defined in terms of words. When an investigator writes a paper or prepares to give a talk, he or she often thinks in terms of words, not pictures. However, since so many of us learn through pictures, visual communication is an important, sometimes essential, and certainly effective way to inform.

An excellent scientist may be famous for wearing unmatched socks. Another may be acutely observant in the laboratory, but could not tell the color of the Golden Gate Bridge. All of us have examples of this phenomenon in and out of science. It is safe to say that we do not see most of the details of our own lives. We are visually unaware.

This book is based on the view that clarification of ideas by visual means, by illustration, is not only effective but can be learned by even the most visually inarticulate.

Good Illustrations

A good illustration can help the scientist to be heard when speaking, to be read when writing. It can help in the sharing of information with other scientists. It can help to convince granting agencies to fund the research. It can help in the teaching of students. It can help to inform the public of the value of the work.

- A good illustration addresses the viewer appropriately. The kind and number of illustrations, the amount of information conveyed, and the level of simplification or complexity of the illustrations should be designed for a specific viewing audience.

- A good illustration supports, enhances, and emphasizes the purpose and the words.

- A good illustration is suitably designed for the intended medium: paper, slide, poster. It is of a legible size, has concise and consistent labels, and uses clear forms and symbols.

- A good illustration has balanced composition and visual impact.

In the following pages are examples and discussion of kinds of pictures to use, good and bad examples, and techniques of making good pictures. The purpose of this book is to help the researcher to become more aware of what communicates visually and to help to improve the quality of visuals used.

Using Words

Below is an example of text describing a process.

The life cycle of the nematode, *Neoaplectana carpocapsae*, begins with the infective juvenile (IJ) stage. The IJs infect insects, usually the larvae, by being eaten or by penetrating some other body orifice. Once inside the insect gut, the IJs penetrate the gut wall and enter the haemocoel. They begin the first-generation reproductive cycle by rapidly growing and developing into the fourth juvenile stage. The fourth-stage juveniles grow, molt, and develop into adults. Adult males and females mate and the first-generation giant females produce as many as 10,000 eggs. The eggs develop into first-stage juveniles which grow, molt, and become second-stage juveniles. Here the nematodes have a choice of repeating the reproductive cycle by growing and molting into third-stage juveniles, or by entering the infective cycle. This fork in the developmental pathway is controlled by population and nutrition. In an underpopulated host larva, development is toward the reproductive cycle. In a crowded host larva, the second-stage juveniles develop into IJs. The IJs migrate from the exhausted larval host and seek new hosts to infect.

How long did it take to read this? Is it clear? Was reading it an easy, rewarding experience? Could the process be visualized as it was read?

Using Pictures

Compare the text above with the figure below.

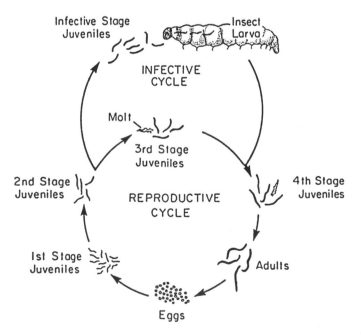

Is this figure more interesting than the text alone? Is it easier to remember? Text and figure together give a fuller understanding than either by itself.

Good ideas do not communicate themselves. Ideas must be organized. Highly complex ideas need to be clarified or simplified while diffuse data may benefit from being combined. Ideas and data must be made interesting and comprehensible to those not familiar with them.

Thorough **planning** is essential and is discussed in the next section. Well-planned and meticulously executed figures are a powerful tool for communication. Figures should be given the same consideration as words.

2

PLAN THE FIGURE

Good planning can save time and money and result in easily understood and interesting figures. Thoughtful planning is perhaps the most important part of an illustration. The most careful drawing and the most expensive execution will not compensate for poor planning. We have all had the experience of being stunned by a blazing color, high-tech slide that leaves us baffled when we try to understand its content.

When to Use a Figure

• Use a figure when words will not suffice. Photomicrographs, tracings (as from electrocardiographs), gels, and anatomical drawings are examples of when a figure is a necessity.

• Use a figure for verisimilitude. Photographs, gels, and tracings are necessary proofs of research findings.

• Use a graph or table to provide the audience with the tools for critical analysis of the work.

• Use a figure to clarify, simplify, and summarize information.

• Use a figure to emphasize information.

• Use a figure to provide background information. Even the sharpest audience appreciates a reminder of what it may already know.

What to Illustrate

- **Anatomy, microanatomy, pathology, and histology** usually require an explanatory drawing, photograph, or diagram. Sometimes photographs of patients are required.

- **Equipment, techniques, and procedures** are most clearly shown in drawings or diagrams.

- **Pathways, schema, and hypotheses** are shown succinctly and simply in flow charts or diagrams.

- **Hypotheses and statements** that need emphasis may be shown in word charts.

- **Tracings and experimental records** are an essential part of communication and are factual verification of research.

- **Data** may be shown in tables, or, more clearly, as graphs. These provide the audience with the means to critically evaluate the experiments.

How Much Information?

The most common disaster in illustrating is to include too much information in one figure. The more points made in an illustration, the more the risk of confusing and discouraging the viewer.

- Slides, posters, and figures in journals are not equivalent in the amount of information presented. A published figure which can be studied may include more information and still be clear. Figures for slides and posters should be simple and uncluttered.

- The amount of information to be presented is determined by the intended viewer. Some viewers have the background to understand more complexities in a subject. Others will comprehend more from several simple figures.

- The amount of information is determined by the medium. Posters are limited by size; slide viewing is limited by time; the printed figure is limited by space and money considerations.

- The amount of information is determined by the novelty or controversial content of the information. To be clear, such information should be presented in the simplest, most uncluttered way.

Find Out About the Viewer

• The viewer's background–such as age, education, and profession–will determine the level of complexity of the figures.

• Some viewers will require more background and explanatory figures. For most viewers drawings and diagrams are more helpful than words and tables.

Know the Media Requirements

• If the figure will be used in a journal paper, instructions to authors should be followed (usually included in one issue per volume). Since these instructions generally have very few guidelines for the presentation of figures, look through the journal to see the style of figures in papers which have been accepted.

• For lectures, consider the size of the room and the kind of projection equipment available. Check that the equipment is working. It is best to project slides ahead of time to avoid the embarrassment of upside-down and backward slides.

• For poster sessions, know the dimensions of the space available. Know the size of the meeting, the location, and the layout of the poster hall, the breadth of your audience's interests, the quality of the lighting, and the amount of space around and between posters.

Plan Integral Figures

• Keep in mind that each figure is a part of a whole context. It must relate to the other parts of the whole.

• Be consistent in format, size, and terminology.

• Avoid repetition except to emphasize.

• Try to create a smooth, logical flow of information with the figures. Often the essence of the information will be clear from the figures alone and extensive explanations are not needed.

Plan For Sufficient Time and Money

Vast amounts of time and money are spent in planning and carrying out experiments. Do not sacrifice this effort by failing to apply the same attention to the presentation of the results.

- Allow time to think carefully about the rough figure. Discuss the figure with others.

- Allow time to revise the rough figure, perhaps more than once.

- Allow time for changes and corrections in the final figure.

- Plan to spend more time and money on drawings and complex figures.

- Allow sufficient time and money for the necessary photography, enlargements, and mounting of the final figure.

Plan to Communicate Visually

In planning illustrations, stand away from the information and imagine the viewer. Think of the information in terms of **what it will look like to another**. Translate the information into visual form.

An Exercise in Planning

The following example uses data associated with the nematode life cycle shown in the previous chapter and reproduced below. Four sets of data from an *in vitro* culture are plotted in the graph to the right of the diagram. The data were collected by inoculating culture vessels with infective juvenile nematodes. The nematodes were harvested and counted at each developmental stage.

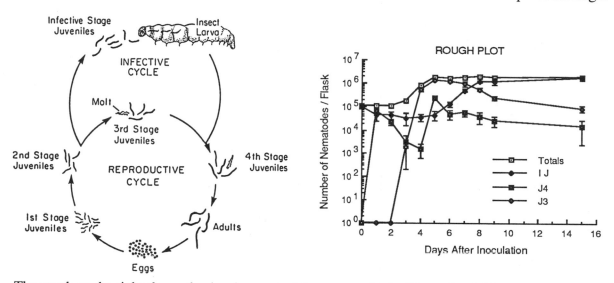

The graph on the right shows the development of three stages in the life cycle of this nematode. The inoculum of infective juveniles changes into 4th stage juveniles, then adults who reproduce. Some of the progeny of this reproduction take the path to 3rd stage juveniles and repeat the reproductive cycle, while others take the path to development of infective juveniles.

The information is clear in the diagram but is a visual thicket of tangled information in the graph. How to make complexities visually clear is what planning is about. There are many ways to do this and the planning process is an opportunity for experimenting with these different ways. On the following pages, the information presented in the graph above is shown in different ways to illustrate some of the options to consider in the planning stage.

The planning stage is the time to approach your information from many angles. Ask yourself, "Will the viewer understand this? Is this the best way to show my information?"

One graph for each set of data is a way to start. They are lined up one above the other to compare the changes over time. For easier comparison, all the scales on the ordinate are plotted as logarithmic scales.

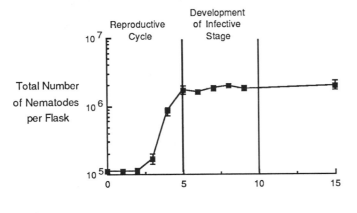

This graph shows that the reproductive cycle lasts about five days.

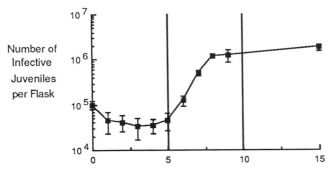

This graph shows that development of new infective juveniles does not begin until after the reproductive cycle.

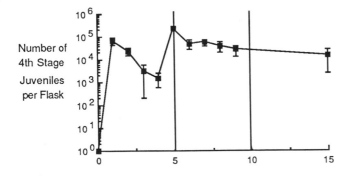

This graph shows two peaks, implying two turns of the life cycle. The first peak results from infective juveniles in the inoculum developing into 4th stage juveniles.

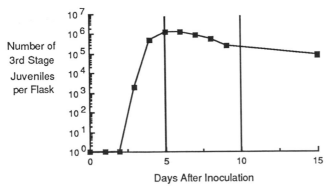

This graph shows that the progeny of the reproductive cycle largely goes into the 3rd juvenile stage. These 3rd stage juveniles develop into the second peak of 4th stage juveniles as the cycle begins its second developmental turn.

Two sets of data graphed together may be a better and more striking way to show comparisons.

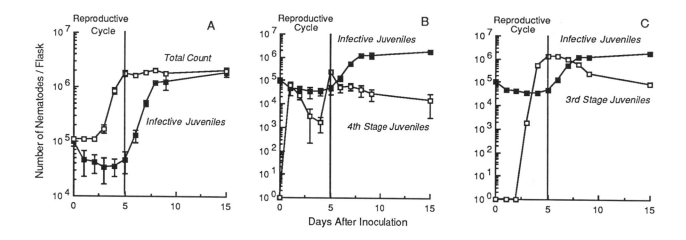

Increase in infective juveniles (A) and the separate paths taken by the 4th and 3rd stage juveniles (B & C) are crucial information. The graphs above clarify these points.

When planning for the best presentation of the data, consider trying other ways and forms to express the information visually.

Scale change and scale limitation is shown in the graph below. The abscissa has been changed from a log to a linear scale. The ordinate stops at 5 days.

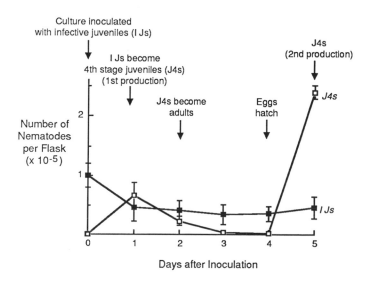

This graph shows changes occurring only during the reproductive cycle and might be a useful background slide to explain the measurements. It serves as a close-up of changes occurring in the first five days.

Try an alternative form. Percentages are shown below as a line graph and a bar graph.

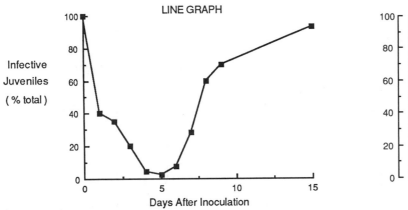

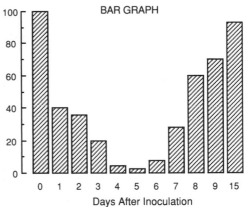

Compare these graphs for their visual message In the line graph, the time of the measurements is evenly spaced and the flow over time is dynamic.The bar graph shows the rise and fall of infected juveniles dramatically and individual measurements are emphasized.

To plan figures effectively:

- Decide on the priorities.
- Clarify and simplify these priorities for the viewer.
- Check for accuracy of expression of these priorities.
- Experiment with different ways to express the information.
- Show the figure to others. Ask them if they understand.

To experiment with different ways to express the information, it is necessary to know the choices. This means having information about the kinds of illustrations available, how to use them effectively, and how to have them made. This means knowledge of the media requirements. The following chapters address these needs.

> The more thoughtfully you plan, the better the figure will be and the more time and money you will save.

3

DRAWINGS AND DIAGRAMS

There are many ways to illustrate scientific and medical information. Sometimes there will be a choice. For instance, should a drawing or a photograph be used to show a laboratory set-up? Should a graph or a table be used to illustrate the data?

In this chapter and the next four chapters are some examples of kinds of illustrations and their appropriate use. "Appropriate" here means fitting the needs to the intended goal. To choose the appropriate illustration, the purpose, audience, and medium must be understood.

When the French artist Edgar Degas stated, "In a single brush stroke, we can say more than a writer in a whole volume," he might have added, "We can say it compellingly and interestingly, too." An appropriate drawing can eliminate pages of text; it can give insights; it can be a vivid and memorable part of the information. In addition to describing succinctly, it can add vigor to the presentation.

On the following pages are examples of a few of the ways in which drawings may be used.

ANATOMICAL DRAWING

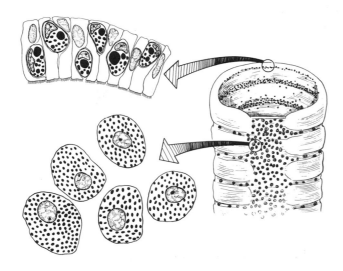

A drawing can simplify anatomical complexities. The line drawing on the left juxtaposes tracheal anatomy with an exploded view of the tracheal cells. This is one advantage a drawing has over a photograph.

MICROANATOMICAL DRAWING

METABOLIC PATHWAYS OF LUNG SURFACTANT

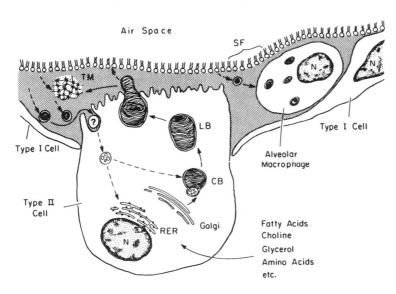

This drawing summarizes elements found in several photomicrographs. By simplification, it emphasizes essential points of microanatomy and clearly identifies those elements. The arrows indicate dynamic movement of the pathways.

PATHOLOGY DRAWING

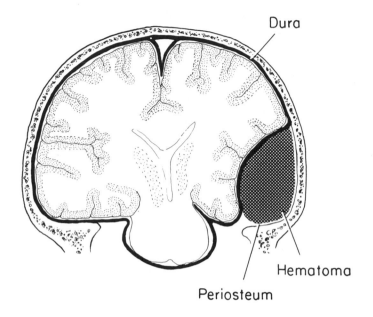

Dura

Hematoma

Periosteum

A drawing is an effective way to emphasize information. Here, attention is called to a cerebral hematoma. The skull and cerebrum are simply outlined, but the areas of interest are darker and textured.

SURGICAL DRAWING

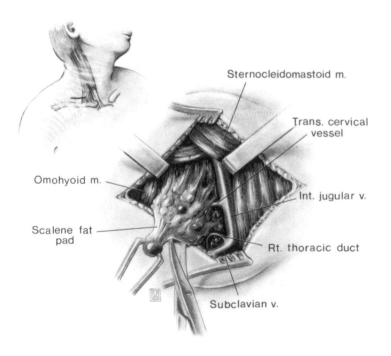

Sternocleidomastoid m.

Trans. cervical vessel

Omohyoid m.

Int. jugular v.

Scalene fat pad

Rt. thoracic duct

Subclavian v.

A drawing of surgery removes possibly disturbing elements. It eliminates distracting background and simplifies and emphasizes information. This drawing shows the isolation of the scalene node more clearly and simply than a photograph. In the head and neck view the muscles of the neck are ghosted under the skin and the line of incision is shown.

TECHNICAL DRAWING

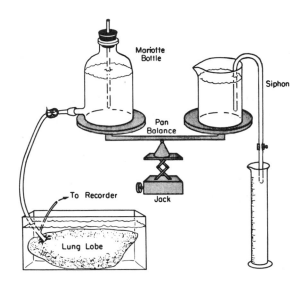

This drawing isolates essential points from a complicated background. Uneven proportions are useful to emphasize one element over another.

DIAGRAM OF ANATOMICAL PATHWAYS

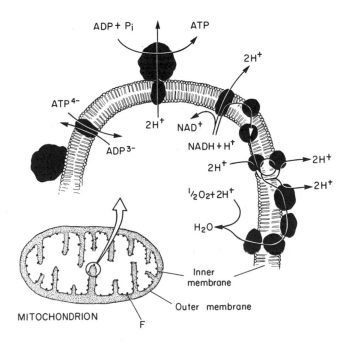

This exploded view of mitochondrial membranes shows dynamic movement of elements across the membranes. Drawings or diagrams are an excellent way to present hypotheses, theories, and imaginative ideas.

DIAGRAM OF EQUIPMENT

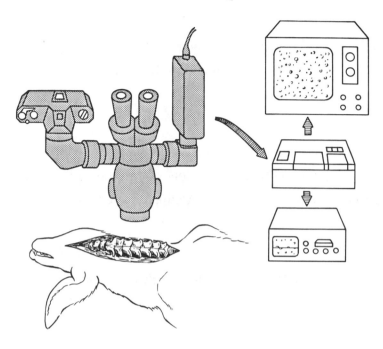

In this diagram, various pieces of equipment are shown together demonstrating the sequence of their use. Showing the equipment with the drawing of the dog trachea makes the orientation immediately clear. This is an effective illustration of experimental method.

SCHEMATIC DIAGRAM

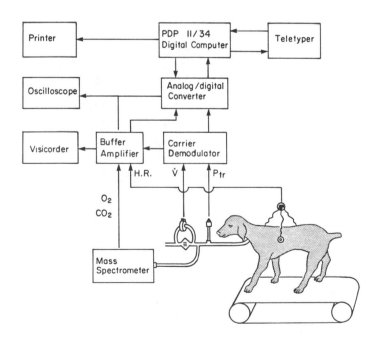

In this drawing, equipment is represented by labeled boxes. The drawing of the dog on the treadmill takes the place of a word box. It explains the procedure more briefly and vividly than words.

Line or Continuous Tone Drawing?

The terms "line" or "continuous tone" are used often in photography and printing and will be discussed in further chapters in that context. In the context of the drawings themselves, the terms refer to the materials and techniques used.

A **line drawing** is done in pen and ink or any other medium which results in black and white only. (Most computer drawings are line drawings.) In a line drawing, tones of grey may be achieved by stippling, fine contour lines, hatching, or cross hatching. A stipple pattern is made up of small black dots.

A **continuous tone** drawing may be done in pencil, watercolor wash, or airbrush. This results in a range of greys. Fine detail and great realism are possible in this technique.

LINE DRAWING   CONTINUOUS TONE DRAWING

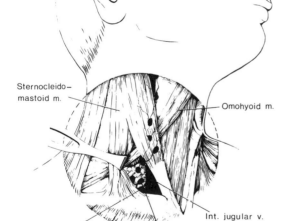
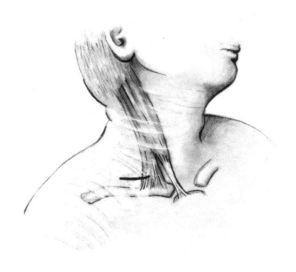

Detail is shown only by lines, and black and white spaces in the line drawing. Grey tone is achieved by lines. The continuous tone drawing was done with carbon pencil and the "dust" or fine scrapings from the pencil brushed on the paper to create tone.

Continuous tone drawings make effective slides because, with enlargement, subtleties and a wide range of tone are preserved. However, for the printing process, the drawings must be converted into an array of tiny dots (half-tone dots). Thus, with reduction to one column of a journal, similar to the reproduction above, some range of tone disappears and the darkest areas might close up and become black.

Fine lines may be lost in a line drawing as well when reduction is great. Care should be taken to be sure lines are sharp and black. Be sure that the dots of any stipple used are large enough not to fade away and well enough spaced not to coalesce or turn to black in reduction.

Communicating With the Artist

In most cases, drawings will be done by an artist. In order for the artist to help communicate the information, the artist needs to know:

- The purpose: the important points of the information.
- The medium: slide, paper, poster.
- How much time he/she will have to do the illustration.

A scientific drawing should be a collaborative effort between author and artist. For this, the artist needs as much understanding of the subject as possible, and the author needs the artist's ideas about presentation. This pooling of ideas is essential to the planning and preparation of a drawing. Be willing to try out new ways to present the information. Since the first stage of a drawing is a sketch, and sketches are easy to change, explore other options at this stage. Take the time to make changes.

Plan more time for a drawing than for other kinds of illustration. Discussion, a sketch (perhaps more than one), revisions, and final drawing all take time. Because of the extra time involved, drawings are more expensive, so be prepared to pay more for a drawing than other kinds of illustration.

Appropriate drawings can communicate faster and more dynamically than words. They clarify, simplify, and emphasize information in an interesting and inspiring way. While they are expensive and time consuming, they will be a priceless help to you in communicating your information.

4

PHOTOGRAPHS

Photographs may be essential for validation and documentation. X-rays, photomicrographs, photographs of patients and specimens are examples.

Photographs are also essential for reproducing figures you have produced.

In illustrating scientific information, photography will be used in two different ways:

1. Reproduction for slide, publication, or poster of the illustration that has been produced by drawing or photography.
2. Production of a figure by photographic means.

While this chapter concentrates on the latter, production of a figure by photographic means, it is important to recognize or review the requirements for good reproduction.

Photographic Reproduction

Good photographic reproduction of drawings or photographic figures can mean the difference between a figure that is clear and legible and one that frustrates because it cannot be seen easily. Responsibility for good reproduction rests with both the author and photographer. For best results, both the author and the photographer should cooperate and be clear about their requirements.

Following are listed some of the requirements of both author and photographer. Keep these in mind while still in the planning stage. It will ultimately save time and money and result in photographs that will enhance the project.

An author requires of the photographer:

- Fidelity to the original. Any enhancement or manipulation must not distort the original.

- Proper enlargement or reduction.

- Good resolution.

- A full tonal range for continuous tone subjects.

- Sharp contrast for black and white subjects.

- A photographer requires of the author:

  - Clear, clean originals.

  - Complete, fully labeled original with complete arrangement of all separate parts.

  - Uniform density of line in the original work.

  - Uniform background for color or continuous tone originals, without paste-ups, cuts, or white outs.

  - Specific and clearly stated directions as to reduction, contrast, grouping of pictures, and emphasis.

  - A format which is appropriate for the medium intended.

For best results, consult the photographer while in the planning stage. Explain to him or her the medium that will be used and the purpose of the figure. A photographer can suggest the size that is most convenient to work with, the format and dimensions of the paper and film being used, and whether a figure may be effectively enlarged or reduced.

If a commercial photographer is used, discussion in the planning stage covering questions, needs, and expectations is especially important. Show the photographer examples of the kind of reproduction you want. If you want to do your own photography, consultation in the planning stage with a professional photographer may be invaluable. To find a photographer who specializes in scientific and medical photography, contact a nearby medical school or hospital.

Tracings

Examples of physiologic tracings illustrate some of the problems in reproducing figures and point out the importance of interaction between photographer and author in solving those problems.

Below are electro-encephalographic tracings which record sleep patterns. They are recorded on paper with a background grid, so that the first decision to make is whether or not to keep the grid. It is possible to eliminate colored grids photographically by using filters. If both grid and tracing are the same color, for example black or red, it is impossible to eliminate the grid. A photographer can easily determine whether the grid can be eliminated.

WITH GRID   WITHOUT GRID

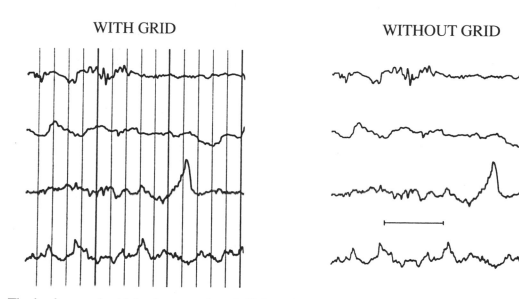

The background grid for these tracings is light red; the tracings are black. In the tracing on the left, the vertical grid marking the tracing time is left in. On the right the grid has been eliminated and a time scale has taken its place. The changes in the tracing patterns are clearer without the grid.

Sometimes tracings are faint and uneven. A photograph or sometimes even a photocopy of the tracing from a copier may darken faint lines and increase the contrast. Try the photocopy machine before consulting the photographer.

The best photographer, however, cannot separate overlapping tracings.

OVERLAPPING TRACINGS

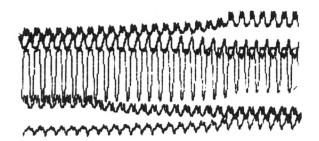

These tracings were set too close together. While an artist could separate them by laboriously redrawing each curve, it would be more efficient to redo the tracing using appropriate settings to separate them.

Settings for tracings should be planned with possible reproduction in mind. Remember this also when **marking tracings**. Do not expect the photographer to touch up or erase thick, indelible notes made on the part of the tracing to be used. To save time, and for better final results, mark the tracing with pencil or mark it above or below the part which will be used.

Selection and mounting of tracings which will be used together is the author's responsibility.

SELECTION AND SEPARATION

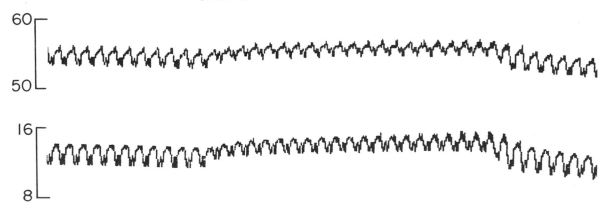

These tracings were parts of larger tracings, selected for their relevance. The light computer print-out was photocopied to darken the lines. Since the left-hand scales overlapped, they were cut apart and mounted with space between them. Scales were redrawn and numbers added by hand.

Use only the parts of the tracing pertaining to the point to be made, keeping in mind the final shape and reduction on the figure. A photographer can assess how effectively the lines will reduce and can advise about format for the medium to be used.

Often many tracings are shown together. Extraneous parts of the tracings must be eliminated and relevant tracings should be placed in a logical order. Repetitious labels should be eliminated and labels added which will fully clarify your information.

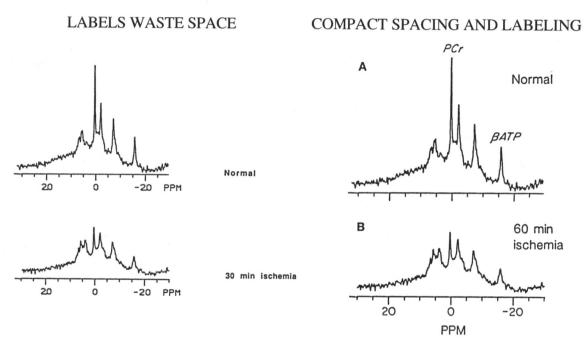

LABELS WASTE SPACE   COMPACT SPACING AND LABELING

There is wasted space and unnecessary repetition of scale numbers in the figure on the left. On the right, repetitious numbers were cut, allowing the tracings to be moved closer together. The more compact arrangement of the labels works well for reduction to one-column journal width. Notice the greater reduction of the figure on the left because of its width. The addition of peak labels and the distinguishing letters, A and B, makes the figure clearer to the viewer and easier to discuss in publication or slide.

Labeling of tracings should be complete and appropriate before submission to a photographer. The style of the labels should be thin-line. Bold or thick labels compete with, and usually overpower, the thin tracing lines. Discuss with the photographer whether it would be better to label a photograph of the tracing or the original tracing.

Photographic Figures

X-rays, photomicrographs, and gels function as data. Photographs from the CRT screens are considered documentation. These photographs give factual information, verisimilitude, or proof.

In addition, photographs may be required of **patients** or **experimental animals** for utmost realism. With patients, it is essential to get their permission and preserve as much of their privacy and anonymity as possible. Although it is not necessary to get permission to use photographs of animals, given the controversial nature of working with animals today, it is wise to avoid photographs showing anything which might be construed as cruel. A selected part of the experimental procedure or a diagrammatic drawing might be a better alternative.

Since "reality" and "truth" are so important in these figures, it is important to be straightforward and thoughtful in the selection of the areas to be used. Manipulation such as enlargement, reduction, increase, or decrease of contrast must not distort or change the information. Touch-up is permissible only to eliminate distracting artifacts. Labels should be used judiciously and sparingly, and should not hide or distract from important information.

In this chapter, examples of photomicrographs, gels, and video images are used to show that clear communication of the information in these photographs requires extensive planning and careful treatment.

Plan Photographs Carefully

- Locate the area of interest near the center of the picture.
- Eliminate unnecessary details.
- Keep the photograph as close to the final reproduction size and/or format as possible.
- Use as few intermediate steps as possible to go from original to reproduction.
- Use thought and care in mounting photographs together.
- Use labels which are proportionate to the size of the photograph.
- Make labels consistent in size and style.

High-Contrast and Continuous Tone Photographs

High-contrast film captures only white and black. It does not record grey tones. Continuous tone film records a full range of tones from white to black.

HIGH-CONTRAST   CONTINUOUS TONE

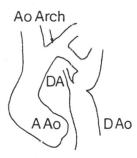

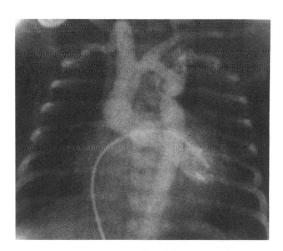

Since the pen and ink drawing on the left includes only black and white tones, it was shot using high-contrast film. The angiogram on the right includes a range of greys and was photographed with continuous tone film.

The advantage of shooting with high-contrast film is that defects in the original such as white-outs and cut-and-paste-lines as in paste-on labels will not show in the final print. Greater care must be taken with the continuous tone original and labeling is best done with a transfer type.

Photomicrographs

Photomicrographs encompass a full tonal range from white to black and are shot with a continuous tone film. Fine, crisp resolution of detail is the goal of these photographs. However, **careful planning** is the essence of their final presentation.

Size of Prints

Before the photomicrograph is printed, know what the final size will be. This is particularly true for journal presentation. There should be no reduction from the print to final reproduction in a journal. Plan the dimensions to fill the column or page in order to avoid wasting space. Plan whether to group images into one figure. Plan the final size to illustrate the main point. Plan whether you will cover your image with labels or show a labeled diagram next to the image.

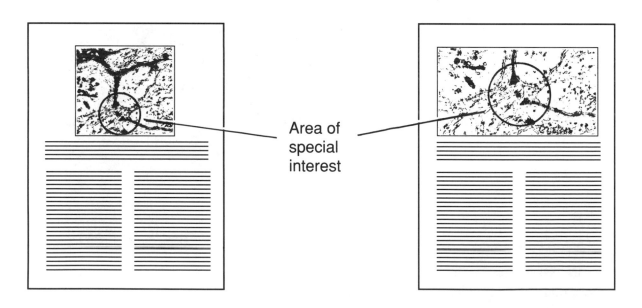

The micrograph on the left leaves empty space around it.. The area of special interest is small and at the bottom of the figure. The figure on the right fills the page space. The area of special interest is centered and enlarged.

Templates For Page Dimensions

Before making final prints, draw a template duplicating the exact page dimensions. Done quickly and in pencil, this will indicate the shape of the final print, how it will fit in the page, and where the legend will be positioned.

PAGE AND FIGURE TEMPLATES

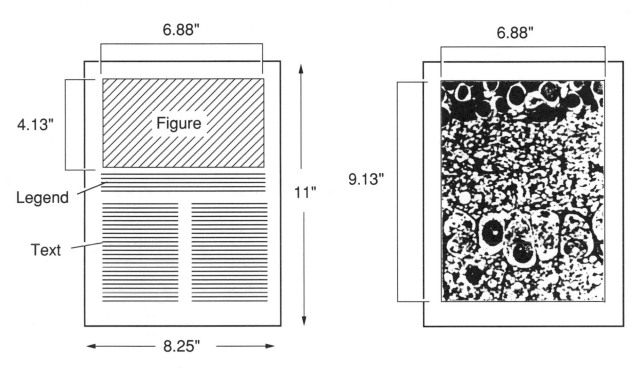

Here, the page and margins are dawn with exact dimensions. On the left, the print is scaled to occupy half of a page with its legend. On the right, a photocopy of the print occupies the whole page without its legend. It is acceptable to put the figure legend at the bottom of the facing page.

Use a template to determine the exact dimensions of the final figure before the print is made. This is especially important when arranging groups of figures. Do not expect the journal to group figures together. This requires time, thought, and experimentation and should be done before making final prints. Determine the focus and magnification for each separate figure on the basis of their relationship to each other. The weighing of priorities, in turn, may be influenced by the space the photographs will occupy.

Arrangement

The grouping of figures should be logical, according to related content. The images to be grouped should not be widely different in tonality. The composition of the grouping should be balanced. Decide ahead of time whether the final figure will be in a one-column space, half page or a full page. If it is to be a slide, decide ahead of time which slide format will be used. The space between the separate figures should not be so great that it will waste space, or appear as a glaring white grid pattern between photographs. However, the space should be large enough to show the figures as clearly separate.

POOR ARRANGEMENT   PLEASING ARRANGEMENTS

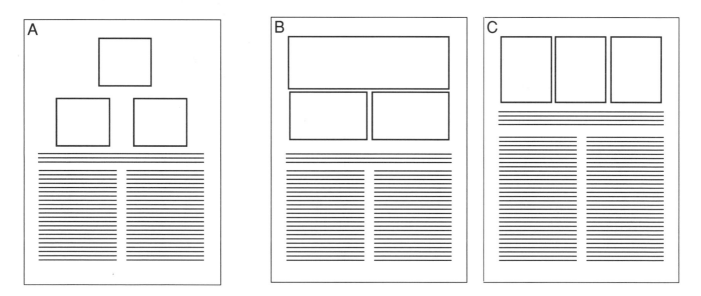

In A, the empty white space gapes and distracts. In a slide, this would be especially pronounced. The relationship between the three photographs is not clear. In the two arrangements on the right, the figures become an integral part of the page, and the eye is led naturally and easily from the photographs to the legend, and on to the text.

The arrangement of three figures together poses special problems. If all three are of equal significance, they should be the same size and placed side by side as in figure C above. If one is clearly more important, it could benefit by expansion and enlargement as in figure B above.

If one figure is clearly subordinate to the other two, consider whether the least important figure could be inset into the figure with which it is most closely related, as below.

FIGURE INSET

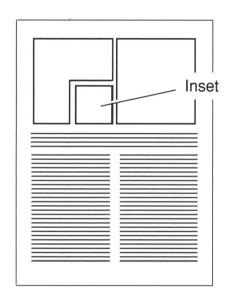

An inset must be carefully planned to fit into the larger figure. It must not obscure essential information. This usually means moving the focus of interest away from the center of the larger photograph. The least conspicuous position for an inset is the lower right-hand corner.

VERTICAL ARRANGEMENT

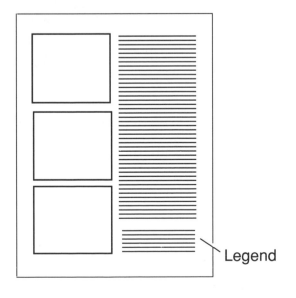

A vertical arrangement of photomicrographs is unusual unless it occupies an entire page. One reason for this is that placement of a legend is awkward in a vertical arrangement. Another reason is that spatial relationship is not so clear, probably because we are accustomed to read from left to right.

For slides, a horizontally rectangular, or square arrangement works best. Many speakers do not label micrographs. Labeling of even large negatives is difficult and not really necessary, since the lecturer can point to and describe the significant areas.

Labels

Labels are secondary to the picture and should be short. They should serve as cues to the explanations in the legend. Labeling should be done directly on the photograph using white or black transfer, or rub-on letters. These may be bought at art supply stores or some stationery stores. Choose a simple font that will not distract. Choose a size which will be legible, and use it consistently. If all your figures are planned for no reduction to final size, the same size labels may be used throughout. Since journal text size is usually 10 point, an 18 point label works well. If in doubt as to the best size, photocopy the image and label the photocopy before the final labeling.

TOO LARGE   WELL-PROPORTIONED

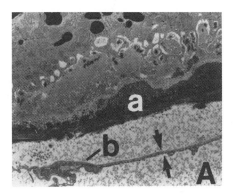   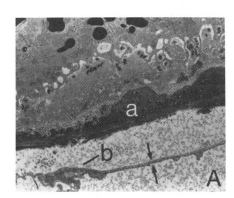

The labels on the left are 24 point Helvetica font in a medium thickness. This size clamors for attention. It is the first thing seen. On the right, the labels are 18 point Helvetica light. They are an integral part of the photomicrograph and inform without distracting. Notice that lower case of the same point size font is smaller than upper case.

One problem with using rub-on labels is that it is easy to run out of the numbers or letters that are frequently used. Be sure to keep a large supply on hand. Another reason for standardizing to one size is to avoid the temptation to use another size in place of the most appropriate size.

Different placement of the labels may be tried first on photocopies. Do not obscure important details with labels. If many labels are essential, consider making a diagram of the image which can then be labeled without cluttering or covering the image.

LABELING BY DIAGRAM

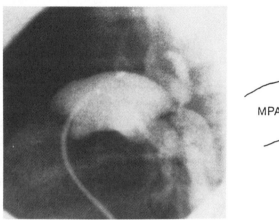 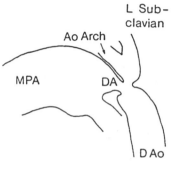

The diagram labels serve to keep the photograph's details clear. The diagram also clarifies structures in the photograph. Both are mounted together to be used as one figure.

A problem in labeling photomicrographs and other continuous tone pictures is whether to use white or black labels. There are times when neither works well. Below are some solutions.

WHITE BACKGROUND LABEL

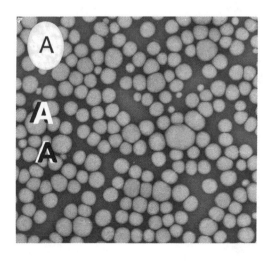

There is no ambiguity about the white background label. These are available in rub-on (transfer) letters, but can be used only as single letters or numbers. Each photo may be labeled with a single number or letter and explained in the legend. Can you find the labels below the white background label? In spite of being outlined by white and black, they disappear into the background.

If labels must be longer than one letter or number, the rub-on labels should be applied to gummed circles or ellipses which have been fixed to the photo. Gummed circles come in different sizes and may be bought in stationery stores.

Arrows and lines are available which are both black and white. These may work best in difficult areas.

LINES AND ARROWS

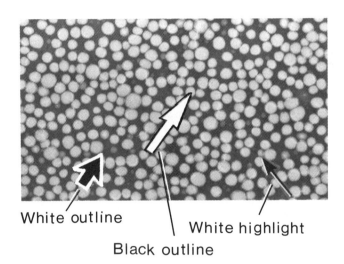

The over-all tonality of this image is neither dark nor light, so that neither black nor white labels show up well. Black rub-on labels are highlighted only on one side. The black arrow outlined thickly with white shows up best. Several styles of arrows are helpful to point out different areas.

White outline

White highlight

Black outline

Consider selecting and cropping prints in such a way that there is a space that is either dark or light enough for labels to show up.

SCALE MARKING

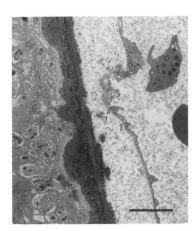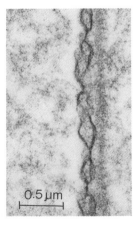

0.5 µm

A scale indicating the magnification must be shown on the photomicrograph. A single, thick line to the exact dimensions (left) is acceptable. In this case, the scale units themselves may be indicated in the figure caption. Or dimensions may be labeled directly on the figure (right). Here the thin scale with end ticks works well against a light background.

Gels

Gel patterns show the array of nucleic acids and proteins separated by electrophoresis into bands of different components, different molecular weights, or restriction fragments. Electrophoresis separates serum proteins into identifiable components. After separation, nucleic acids and proteins may be stained and quantified.

Gel electrophoresis is a powerful analytical tool and is widely used in genetic and peptide mapping. The photography and labeling of gels require special consideration. A light background is desirable with contrast between the darker and lighter bands. Labeling should be legible but unobtrusive.

UNLABELED GEL

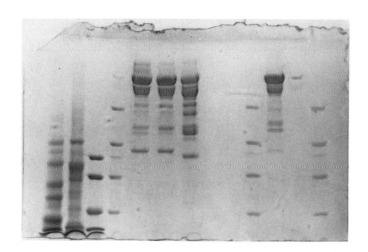

Molecular weight of proteins is assessed in this polyacrylamide gel electrophorcsis using a sodium dodecylsulfate buffer (SDS-PAGE). The wet gel was photographed on a light box using a fine grain film. Good contrast was achieved by experimentally adjusting exposure and time, and by manipulation in printing. This gel was made by Geri Chen, and photographed by David Hardman for Cardiovascular Research Institute, University of California, San Francisco.

A problem in the reproduction of gels is that there may be a slight loss of quality (degradation) with each photographic step away from the original. Labelling must be done on a photographic print of the gel. A negative and print of this print must be made to satisfy most journal requirements for several glossy prints. Then the printer makes another negative and print for publication. Thus, it is most important to have a crisp, sharp first print.

Also, it is advisable to send the original labeled print to the journal. The journal can then make a negative and print from the original. Photographic prints of the original labeled print may also be sent to the journal for use of the reviewers.

Labels will not always fit on the photographic print of the gel. The white surrounding area of the print is usually not wide enough for labels, and labels on the print itself may cover important information. In this case, trim and mount the gel print on white backing paper or board. Trimming and mounting may be done at this time to rearrange, add, or eliminate gel sections.

LABELED GEL

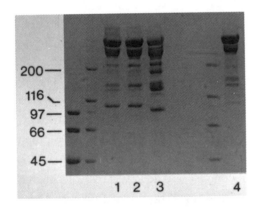

The labels on this gel are 10 point size. The style is simple, sans serif, and thin lined. It is legible but does not distract from the subtle tones of the gel bands.

In the original labeled print, the labels are high-contrast (black and white only) while the gel is continuous tone (containing shades of grey). However, in the reproduction shown above, everything is continuous tone; the background to the labeling is grey. If separate negatives are made of the gel and the surrounding labels, the result is more like the original. This is more time consuming for the photographer, but it results in a clearer, crisper final reproduction (opposite).

GEL PRINTED FROM TWO NEGATIVES

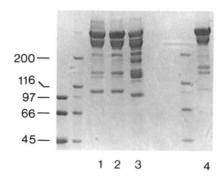

Printing of this figure was done from two negatives. Notice that the background for the labels is pure white, while the gel itself contains a range of greys.

The same standards for label size and thickness apply also to **immunoblots**. For immunoblots, the gel is transfered onto a nitrocellulose filter where it is subjected to a complex of protein antigens and antibodies. It is then exposed to X-ray or to a dye. A print may be made of this and then labeled, or, better yet, labeling may be done directly on the film. If trimming and rearrangement of the columns is necessary, the film may be cut and taped to a clear acetate backing which may then be labeled.

In using transfer labels, stay away from decorative or complicated script types. Choose instead a plain, sans serif type face such as Helvetica. Make sure that you have enough of the correctly sized letters so that you will not have to use an inappropriate size or font.

Video Images

Photographs are often taken from video screens. Echocardiography, ultrasound images, computed tomography, scintigraphy, nuclear magnetic resonance imaging, and others are photographed from the cathode ray tube (CRT) screen. Their effectiveness depends upon the resolution of the screen, the ability to enlarge crucial areas, and the labeling options that the computer program offers.

Below is an example of ultrasound imaging as it comes from the computer screen.

UNIMPROVED

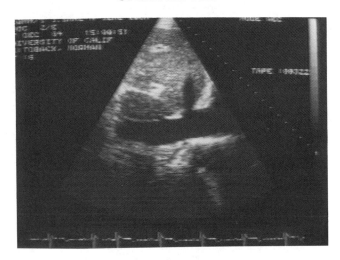

This is an echocardiograph (ECG) showing sections of the inferior vena cava and the hepatic vein. The background labeling (illegible at this reduction) includes the mode, the tape number, the place, patient name and date. At the bottom is an ECG tracing. While this is vital information to the researcher, it is usually irrelevant to the point to be made and should be left. out.

Since most equipment does not allow for changes on the screen, cropping and labeling must be done on the print.

IMPROVED

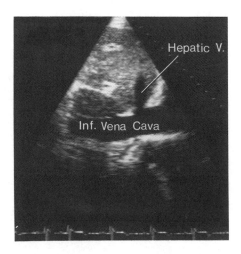

This is the same image. It has been cropped on the sides and the background labels have been blocked. White transfer labels have been applied directly to the print. The ECG tracing has been left in.

The fan shape of the echocardiogram is lost in the black background of the figures on the opposite page. If it is not necessary to include the ECG tracing, a clearer, crisper result is attained by the following method.

REMOVE THE BACKGROUND

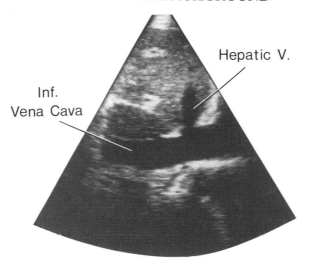

Hepatic V.

Inf.
Vena Cava

The fan shaped echocardiogram was cut from its black background as an easy way of eliminating unwanted background labeling and lines. The black labels on a white background are crisp and clean.

It may not be possible to program the equipment to eliminate or enlarge labels, or to enlarge certain areas and eliminate others. This usually must be done by hand. While it takes a little more time to do this, it may make the difference between communicating or confusing.

In *Chapter 14, Drawing By Hand*, simple processes for trimming, mounting, and labeling tracings and gels are described.

5
CHARTS AND TABLES

Very often the same data can be presented as either a chart or a table. A **chart** contains pictures, words, or numbers, and is outlined or mapped to show sequences, deviations, and pathways. A **table** is a compilation of numerical or alphabetical data arranged in tabulated and labeled columns showing summaries of findings.

Both charts and tables can be effective vehicles for communication. In fact, they are essential for expressing certain kinds of information. Cycles, algorithms, and genealogies must be shown as charts. Essential numerical values and lists of facts to be compared must be shown in tables.

Charts

A good chart delineates and organizes information. It communicates complex ideas, procedures, and lists of facts by simplifying, grouping, and by setting and marking priorities. By spatial organization, it should lead the eye through information smoothly and efficiently.

Below are the steps of the nematode life cycle shown in Chapter 1 simply listed, and then organized into a chart.

LIFE CYCLE LIST   LIFE CYCLE CHART

Infective cycle:

    1. Infective stage juvenile

    2. Infection of insect larva

Reproductive cycle:

    3. Fourth stage juvenile

    4. Adult

    5. Egg

    6. First stage juvenile

    7. Second stage juvenile

    8. Third stage juvenile

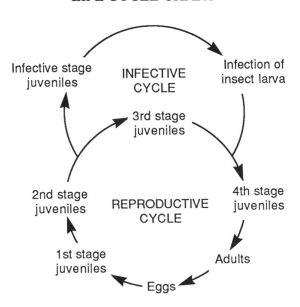

The chart, because of its circular organization, is immediately apparent as a cycle. The relations of the two main divisions, infection and reproduction, are immediately clear. The split path from second stage juvenile to third or infective stage is clearly shown in the chart. In the same amount of space, the chart is more informative and visually more interesting.

It can be made even more informative and interesting by adding simple drawings.

LIFE CYCLE WITH DRAWINGS

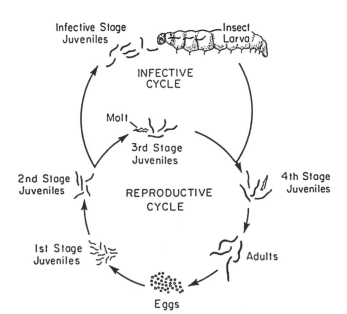

The drawings with the words immediately orient the viewer, refresh the memory, or introduce morphological information. The drawings invite the viewer to pause, look, and consider.

In the following circuit chart of retrograde aortic perfusion, the drawing of the heart actually takes the place of the word, "heart". This is possible only if the subject is immediately familiar and recognizable. The boxing in of words sets them apart and suggests the simplified representation of the labeled entities.

CIRCULAR ARRANGEMENT
WITH BOXES

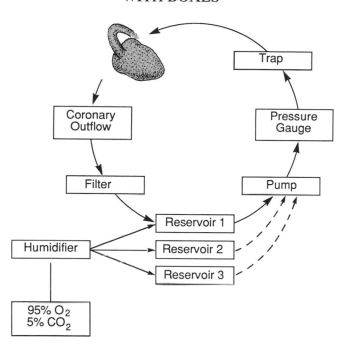

Here, the circuit is shown as circular. The eye is drawn to the heart drawing first as the place to start. The arrows then lead the eye through the heart perfusion. The circular organization emphasizes motion through the system and clearly separates the perfusion cycle from the reservoir components. The boxes symbolize equipment through which the blood passes.

RECTANGULAR ARRANGEMENT

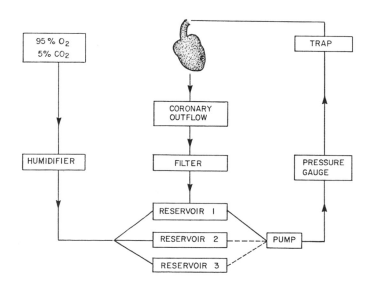

The rectangular arrangement has a neat and pleasing symmetry, but the sense of circular flow is lost. This organization also emphasizes the oxygen / carbon dioxide infusion and the three reservoirs.

A schema presents constituents in a pattern or plan.

SCHEMA OF LUNG INNERVATION

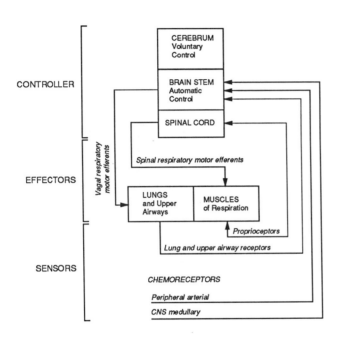

This outline of a system of neural activity groups separately boxed components. The division into three main sections is on the left, and varied size and style of labels set priorities of importance. Movement through the system is directed by arrows.

To communicate, a chart must be carefully organized. Make several rough sketches with different arrangements, keeping in mind the purpose and priorities. Keep it simple: do not put too much information in it. Pool ideas with colleagues, and try to make the chart interesting as well as informative. Make use of boxes or circles, simple drawings, arrows, and varieties of size and style of labels.

> To be effective, both charts and tables must be clearly and simply organized.

Tables

Tables, like dictionaries, are indispensable in our lives. What would we do without the table of measurements, the table of contents, the tide table, the train schedule? We all refer to them from time to time for specific information. However, we do not regard them as entertaining, and we do not read through a whole table unless we have to.

Tables for scientific research are often necessary for looking up specific facts. While they are not the most interesting reading, good, pleasing design with symmetry, balance, and variety invite the reader to look. Good design can help the reader to find information quickly. Disorganized, poorly designed tables are irritating and visually distressing.

A successful table organizes alphabetical or numerical information into columns and rows that are accurate, logical, and easy to follow and understand. Headings should be plain English and unabbreviated. We should be able to read the table without a magnifying glass.

Use a Table:
- To summarize research findings.
- To group together specific data sets to compare and relate.
- To document an account of experimental procedure and results.
- To enable the reader to make calculations from experimental data.
- To enable the reader to reproduce the experiment.

The last two uses for tables, calculation and reproduction of data, although the most important in the larger objective of science, are only useful in published tables. Tables for slides and posters do not allow time for calculation or reproduction uses. Also, because of the short viewing time, tables for posters and slides should contain much less information than those for publication.

Criteria for a Good Table

- A table must be **complete**; i.e., it must be understandable without detailed reference to the text.
- Use **units** that are complete and easily understood.
- The data in a table must be not only accurate, but **pertinent** and **significant**. Select the important aspects of the information.
- Keep the format **clear and simple**. Do not waste space, and be **consistent** in style and terminology.
- Make groupings **logical**.
- Design the table to **fit the format** of a slide, page or poster.

Consider how the viewer will use the information in the table. If the table might be used for calculation or duplication to extend the reader's own work, be sure all data for that purpose are included. For example, recently an attack was made on the work of two researchers, citing, among other things, the inapproriate choice of statistical analysis and the unavailability of raw data.[*] Present pertinent raw data rather than the statistics derived from them.

However, if the table is being used to make comparisons or as a summary, be more selective about the information.

The table on the opposite page is complete enough for calculation or possible duplication. It is taken from a journal, and it contains raw data from experiments with five lambs without kidneys (anephric lambs). Calculations have been made to derive the P values; units are complete and described in the footnotes. It contains a large amount of information and is complete enough for calculation or duplication.

---

[*] Research News. Conflict over DNA clock results. Science 241: 1598–1600. (1988)

JOURNAL TABLE

TABLE V

Pulmonary Hemodynamics and Fluid and Protein Transport in Five Anephric, Anesthetized 1–2-Wk-Old Lambs before and after Intravenous Furosemide, 8 mg/kg

	Weight		Time relative to furosemide infusion	Vascular pressures		Protein concentrations				Lymph flow	Protein flow
	Body	Dry bloodless lung				Lymph		Plasma			
Lamb				$\hat{P}$pa	$\hat{P}$la	Total	% Alb*	Total	% Alb*		
	kg	*g*		*torr*		*g/dl*		*g/dl*		*ml/h·g‡*	*mg/h·g·g_p§*
15	7.3	19.7	Before	17	7	2.90	55	3.90	49	0.11	0.79
			After	17	7	2.83	55	4.04	47	0.09	0.63
16	6.9	18.9	Before	17	8	2.70	48	4.01	45	0.10	0.66
			After	17	9	2.57	53	3.96	44	0.08	0.51
17	5.4	18.0	Before	21	7	2.40	50	4.03	47	0.10	0.62
			After	21	7	2.60	46	4.19	43	0.08	0.49
18	10.0	24.6	Before	25	−1	2.14	55	3.78	47	0.12	0.65
			After	27	1	2.26	54	3.92	48	0.11	0.62
19	5.2	15.5	Before	21	3	1.95	64	3.78	52	0.17	0.88
			After	21	3	1.91	65	3.76	52	0.15	0.77
Mean±SEM	7.0±0.9	19.3±1.5	Before	20±1	5±2	2.42±0.17	54±3	3.90±0.05	48±1	0.12±0.01	0.72±0.05
			After	21±2	5±1	2.43±0.16	55±3	3.97±0.07	47±2	0.10±0.01	0.60±0.05
P				NS	NS	NS	NS	NS	NS	< 0.05	<0.05

* Percent of total protein concentration which is albumin.
‡ Lymph flow relative to dry bloodless lung tissue.
§ Protein flow (lymph flow × lymph protein concentration) relative to dry bloodless lung tissue and plasma protein concentration.

Horizontal lines divide the title, headings, and footnotes from the body of the table. Complex subheadings are also separated by horizontal lines. The means and P values are shown below the data. The journal typeset the table to fit exactly into the width of a page, and the style and size of the text were also specified by the journal.

The table format shown above is standard for most journals. Occasionally, some horizontal lines may be thicker or doubled, but vertical division lines are rarely used. Uniform label size is used throughout the table and is usually the same size as the text except when the table is so large it must be reduced. In this table, lettering size is small enough to cause squinting. In addition, the complexity of heading and units of measurement make this a difficult table in which to find specific information. See the next page for a simplified version of this table.

In the table below, the lamb numbers and weights have been omitted for simplification. Yet it is still complete enough for calculation and reproduction to be made from it. This table also conforms to the journal format.

SIMPLIFIED TABLE FOR A JOURNAL

Data Related to Lung Fluid Balance in Five Anephric, Anesthetized 1-2-wk old Lambs
Before and After Furosemide

Intravenous Furosemide 8 mg / kg	VASCULAR PRESSURES		PROTEIN CONCENTRATIONS				FLOW	
			Lymph		Plasma			Lymph
	Ppa**	Pla***	Total	% Alb	Total	% Alb.	%Lymph	Protein
	Torr		g / dl		g / dl		ml / h g †	mg/h g g_p ‡
Before	17	7	2.90	55	3.90	49	0.11	0.79
After	17	7	2.83	55	4.04	47	0.09	0.63
Before	17	8	2.70	48	4.01	45	0.10	0.66
After	17	9	2.57	53	3.96	44	0.08	0.51
Before	21	7	2.40	50	4.03	47	0.10	0.62
After	21	7	2.60	46	4.19	43	0.08	0.49
Before	25	-1	2.14	55	3.78	47	0.12	0.65
After	27	1	2.26	54	3.92	48	0.11	0.62
Before	21	3	1.95	64	3.78	52	0.17	0.88
After	21	3	1.91	65	3.76	52	0.15	0.77
MEAN ± SEM								
Before	20 ± 1	5 ± 2	2.42 ± 0.17	54 ± 3	3.90 ± 0.05	48 ± 1	0.12 ± 0.01	0.72 ± 0.05
After	21 ± 2	5 ± 1	2.43 ± 0.16	55 ± 3	3.97 ± 0.07	47 ± 2	0.10 ± 0.01*	0.60± 0.05*

* $P < 0.05$ **Ppa = mean pulmonary arterial pressure   ***Pla = mean left atrail pressure
† Relative to dry bloodless lung tissue
‡ Lymph flow x lymph protein concentration / plasma protein concentration, relative to dry bloodless lung tissue

Information for tables should be simplified as much as possible. Leave out data that have no bearing on the point you want to make. Here, the range or means of the lamb weights could be stated in one sentence. The P values are indicated by asterisks. The values without asterisks, by implication, are not significant. Some information in the title has been moved to the heading and the units are put directly under the headings which they describe. Lettering is larger and easier to read.

The table is submitted to a journal in typewritten form and the journal resets it in its own format for publication. If you feel it helps your information to use a different format, you could and should request this. Below is the same table in a format that does not conform to the journal's specifications but which has clearer divisions, making it easier to locate data.

CLEARLY ORGANIZED TABLE

Data Related to Lung Fluid Balance in Five Anephric, Anesthetized 1-2-wk old Lambs
Before and After Furosemide

Intravenous Furosemide 8 mg / kg	VASCULAR PRESSURES		PROTEIN CONCENTRATIONS				FLOW	
			Lymph		Plasma			Lymph
	Ppa	Pla	Total	% Alb	Total	% Alb.	%Lymph	Protein
	Torr		g / dl		g / dl		ml / h g †	mg/h g g_p ‡
Before	17	7	2.90	55	3.90	49	0.11	0.79
After	17	7	2.83	55	4.04	47	0.09	0.63
Before	17	8	2.70	48	4.01	45	0.10	0.66
After	17	9	2.57	53	3.96	44	0.08	0.51
Before	21	7	2.40	50	4.03	47	0.10	0.62
After	21	7	2.60	46	4.19	43	0.08	0.49
Before	25	1	2.14	55	3.78	47	0.12	0.65
After	27	1	2.26	54	3.92	48	0.11	0.62
Before	21	3	1.95	64	3.78	52	0.17	0.88
After	21	3	1.91	65	3.76	52	0.15	0.77
MEAN ± SEM								
Before	20 ± 1	5 ± 2	2.42 ± 0.17	54 ± 3	3.90 ± 0.05	48 ± 1	0.12 ± 0.01	0.72 ± 0.05
After	21 ± 2	5 ± 1	2.43 ± 0.16	55 ± 3	3.97 ± 0.07	47 ± 2	0.10 ± 0.01*	0.60± 0.05*

* $P < 0.05$
† Relative to dry bloodless lung tissue
‡ Lymph flow x lymph protein concentration / plasma protein concentration, relative to dry bloodless lung tissue

The use of vertical lines clarifies the divisions, and the use of upper case and bold lettering sets unambiguous priorities of headings and subheadings. In a table as complicated as this one, use every means possible to clarify the information.

Unfortunately, a request to use a different format may not be granted by the journal. If such is the case, more information might be eliminated so that, even in conformance with the journal standards, the table will be easy to understand.

When simplifying by eliminating information, consider carefully the purpose of the table. If the intention is to summarize findings, the use of means and standard errors would be most effective. If the findings are to be compared and related, use only the pertinent data sets. Be selective about the number of data sets if documentation or facilitation of calculation is the goal. For reproduction of the experiment, two or more tables may be better than one if the information is long and complicated.

Changing a Table Into a Slide

The conclusions to be drawn from the above tables, as stated in the text of the paper, are that while pressures and concentrations do not change, lymph flow decreases by 17% in lambs without kidneys (anephric lambs).

For a slide, these conclusions must be emphasized and the table must be further simplified. It is easier to see that protein concentrations are the same without the albumin data. Also, unless each of the five lamb studies will be discussed separately, it is more effective to show the mean values only. It is here that the significance of the decrease in flow is most evident.

For best results, the table should be completely redesigned for use as a slide (opposite page). The means and standard errors, only, are used. The change in lymph flow is emphasized by eliminating lymph protein flow and by making lymph flow the first column. Since we read from left to right, the first column on the left is the most prominent.

TABLE FOR A SLIDE

LYMPH FLOW DECREASES IN ANEPHRIC LAMBS AFTER FUROSEMIDE

Intravenous Furosemide 8 mg / kg	LYMPH FLOW ml / h g	VASCULAR PRESSURES		PROTEIN CONCENTRATIONS	
		Ppa	Pla	Lymph	Plasma
		Torr		g / dl	
BEFORE	0.12 ± 0.01	20 ± 1	5 ± 2	2.42 ± 0.17	3.90 ± 0.05
AFTER	0.10* ± 0.01	21 ± 2	5 ± 1	2.43 ± 0.16	3.97 ± 0.07

* $P < 0.05$

By cutting out all but the essential information, the text in the slide will be larger and easier to see. The title is changed and abbreviated to state the most important conclusion. The standard errors have been put below the means to conform better to the slide format. The speaker could explain the lymph protein units if necessary. Avoid footnotes in a slide.

Keep in mind that a slide is on the screen for a short time. Use this limited time to communicate the most important facts.

> For a slide of a table, use only concise and pertinent information.

It is not unusual to see a lecture slide of a table, probably taken from a journal, which is so full of miniscule text that it might as well be hieroglyphics. The lecturer then proceeds to tell us to disregard most of the table and to concentrate on one part (which we cannot see). The result is boredom and/or irritation. If a table must be used in a talk, take the time to design one which can easily be seen and understood.

However, for a talk, it might be more concise and informative to design a **graph** which would show the significant observations. (The fact that there was no change in pressure and concentration may be said in one sentence.) Two observations could be illustrated in one graph. First, lymph flow decreased in lambs with no kidneys: second, lymph flow decrease was greater in unanesthetized lambs with kidneys. This last observation was detailed in a separate table in the journal publication.

GRAPH OR TABLE?

DECREASE IN FLOW AFTER FUROSEMIDE INFUSION

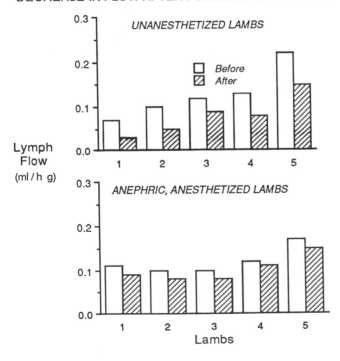

In this graph, two points from the previous table are illustrated:

1.) **Lymph flow decrease** after furosemide is shown by the before and after bars.

2.) **Greater decrease of flow in unanesthetized lambs** is clear in comparing the top and bottom graphs. Five experiments were done with both groups, and it can be seen that there was less lymph flow in general among the anephric lambs.

Tables, especially complex tables, are not effective slides. Think carefully about how you want to present the information, and before making final decisions, experiment with different forms and different ways to organize. Above all, be clear about what you want to communicate in your table.

Consider the possibility of using a drawing with a table. If the data relate to anatomical areas as in the following table, values will be quickly associated and remembered more easily.

TABLE WITH DRAWING

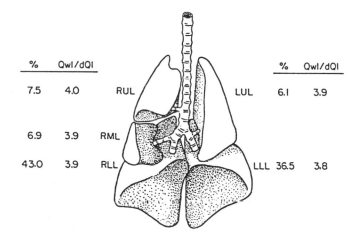

LOBE WEIGHTS AND WATER CONTENT
IN NORMAL SHEEP

%	Qwl/dQl			%	Qwl/dQl
7.5	4.0	RUL	LUL	6.1	3.9
6.9	3.9	RML			
43.0	3.9	RLL	LLL 36.5	3.8	

Flow data are shown next to the different lung lobes from which they were taken. The amount of information is limited and the organization is simple and easily read vertically or horizontally.

The greatest pitfall in designing tables is to include too much information   A page or screen full of lists is daunting and discouraging to the viewer and is not helpful in communicating. Every table can benefit from discriminating selection and cutting.

To Condense Large Tables:

- Remove unnecessary rows and columns. Select the important columns and cut the rest.

- Combine columns which are closely related by using slashes or dashes. For instance, the separate columns, Total Protein and % Albumin in protein could become Total / % Albumin. The data under that heading would then be written 2.90 / 55.

- Do not repeat data that are already in the text or in another table. Do not repeat label information in the heading which may already be in the title or footnote.

Before making a table, ask yourself if it is absolutely necessary. Could that information be said in a few sentences in the text? Could that information be made into a graph? If a table is necessary, limit the amount of information in it and organize it carefully.

6

MOLECULAR GRAPHICS

The story told by molecular structure is still new, exciting, and full of mystery and challenge. Graphical representation of sequences of nucleotides in DNA and RNA, and of amino acids in proteins, and the stereoscopic display of their structure, has played a crucial part in understanding, as well as communicating the subject. The graphics used in biochemical study represent sequences, sequence alignment and folding, maps of nucleic acid sequence restriction sites, and models of molecular structure.

In this chapter, the focus will be on black and white representation of the graphics because that is still most widely used in journals and slides. Color, however, is so helpful in clarifying the complexities of models, in particular, that a discussion of its use is also included.

Genetic Sequences

A sequence is a code for the components in the long chain of molecules. As new sequences are determined, these data may be fed into a computer. Computer programs have been developed to order sequences of nucleic acid bases, and to translate DNA and RNA sequences into amino acids. Programs have been designed to find homology and consensus in aligning different sequences, and to locate patterns or motifs. Possibilities for the folding of the polypeptide chains may be displayed, and sites for enzyme cutting or restriction may be mapped.

Sophisticated computer programs have been developed for analyzing and displaying molecular sequences. Not only do such programs digest and analyze great quantities of sequence information, they do it rapidly and accurately. Judging from journals, the use of such programs is widespread.

Although these programs are vital for learning, they are not always designed for effective communication. Computer-printed figures from such programs are rarely effective for publication, slide, or poster because they are too small to be read, too complex to be understood, and the wrong shape to fit the medium used. The following examples suggest ways to modify computer-printed sequences in order to communicate more effectively.

Because its basic form is a string of letters like a cryptogram, a sequence is more like text than pictures. However, here it is included under graphics because of the graphical elements used to clarify it.

TRANSLATED SEQUENCE

```
-35             -30
Asn Thr Thr Thr Gly Glu Ser Ala Asp Pro Val Thr Thr Thr Val
AAC ACT ACC ACC GGG GAG TCT GCA GAC CCT GTC ACC ACC ACC GTT

-20                           -10
Glu Asn Tyr Gly Gly Glu Thr Gln Val Gln Arg Arg Gln His Thr
GAA AAC TAC GGC GGT GAG ACA CAA GTC CAA CGA CGT CAG CAC ACC

            1                               10
Asp Val Thr Phe Ile Met Asp Arg Phe Val Lys Ile Gln Asn Leu
GAC GTT ACT TTC ATA ATG GAC AGA TTT GTA AAG ATA CAA AAT TTG

                        20
Asn Pro Ile His Val Ile Asp Leu Met Gln Thr His Gln His Gly
AAC CCC ATA CAT GTC ATT GAC CTC ATG CAA ACC CAC CAA CAC GGG

            30                          40
Leu Val Gly Ala Leu Leu Arg Ala Ala Thr Tyr Tyr Phe Ser Asp
TTG GTA GGT GCC CTG TTA CGT GCT GCT ACG TAC TAC TTC TCT GAC

                    50
Leu Glu Ile Leu Val Arg His Asp Gly Asn Leu Thr Trp Val Pro
CTG GAG ATT CTG GTA CGC CAT GAC GGT AAC CTA ACC TGG GTA CCC

                60                          70
Asn Gly Ala Pro Glu Ala Ala Leu Ser Asn Met Gly Asn Pro Thr
AAC GGA GCA CCC GAG GCA GCT CTG TCT AAC ATG GGC AAC CCC ACC

                    80
Ala Tyr Pro Lys Ala Pro Phe Thr Arg Leu Ala Leu Pro Tyr Thr
GCC TAC CCC AAG GCA CCA TTT ACG AGG CTC GCG CTC CCC TAC ACC

            90                          100
Ala Pro His Arg Val Leu Ala Thr Val Tyr Asn Gly Thr Ser Lys
GCG CCA CAC CGC GTA TTG GCG ACA GTG TAC AAC GGG ACG AGC AAG

                    110
Tyr Ser Ala Gly Gly Met Gly Arg Arg Gly Asp Leu Glu Pro Leu
TAC TCC GCA GGT GGT ATG GGC AGA CGG GGC GAC CTA GAG CCT CTC

            120                         130
Ala Ala Arg Val Ala Ala Gln Leu Pro Thr Ser Phe Asn Phe Gly
GCG GCG AGG GTC GCC GCT CAG CTT CCT ACT TCT TTC AAC TTT GGT

                    140
Ala Ile Gln Ala Thr Thr Ile His Glu Leu Leu Val Arg Met Lys
GCA ATT CAA GCC ACG ACC ATC CAC GAG CTC CTC GTG CGC ATG AAG
```

On the left is part of a DNA alpha 22 sequence with its translation from nucleotide base to amino acid residue. Each amino acid is separated by a space and every tenth one is numbered. It has been reduced to the size of one journal column.

The sequence shown above is a working blueprint. From it can be discovered the number and length of repeated motifs and the sites at which DNA cutting enzymes may act. It is a tool for working and deduction. In its raw form, however, it discourages communication. The explanation for such a figure would take a great deal of space and time.

If it is necessary to show a whole sequence, treat it as an orientation map, pointing to areas of interest. Expand the areas of interest in additional figures. This may mean transferring the sequence, or part of the sequence, to a computer drawing program with options for selection, enlargement, addition of lines, boxes, and patterns. While this takes time and thought, if it gets the message across, it will be worth it.

Following are suggestions for clarifying and simplifying:

The choices of font change and change of letter size are usually not options in the computer printed sequences. The sequence requires a font that is evenly spaced, like Courier, rather than a proportionally spaced font like Times, since the alignment of letters one above the other must be exact. Enlargement of letter size of a long sequence without cutting or simplifying it will make no difference in its final reduction since the sequence size is still the same.

Spacing, however, is an important option to consider. The following examples show numbering and spacing that may enhance readability.

UNSPACED

```
CTGCAGGCTCAAAAATGACCAGGCTAACTA
GACGTCCGAGTTTTTACTGGTCCGATTGAT

CTCGCTCAACACAGATGACCCGCTCATCTT
GAGCTAGTTGTGTCTACTGGGCCGGTAGAA

CAAGTCCACCCTGGACACTGATTACCAGAT
GTTCACGTGGGACCTGTGACTAATGGTCTA

GACCAAACGGGACATGGGCTTTACTGAAGA
CTGGTTTGCCCTGTACCCGAAATGACTTCT

GGAGTTTAAAAGGCTGGTGAGTGG
CCTCAAATTTTCCGACCACTCAGG
```

SPACED AND NUMBERED

```
         10         20         30
CTGCAGGCTC AAAAATGACC AGGCTAACTA
GACGTCCGAG TTTTTACTGG TCCGATTGAT

         40         50         60
CTCGCTCAAC ACAGATGACC CGCTCATCTT
GAGCTAGTTG TGTCTACTGG GCGAGTAGAA

         70         80         90
CAAGTCCACC CTGGACACTG ATTACCAGAT
GTTCAGGTGG GACCTGTGAC TAATGGTCTA

        100        110        120
GACCAAACGGG ACATGGGCT TTACTGAAGA
CTGGTTTGCCC TGTACCCGA AATGACTTCT

        130        140
AGGAGTTTAA AGGCTGGTGA GTGG
TCCTCAAATT TCCGACCACT CACC
```

Both figures show paired bases of human adenosine deaminase. There is no easy way to discuss components of the unspaced figure on the left. Finding individual units in the spaced and numbered figure on the right is much less difficult. Note that the spacing between the lines clearly separates the grouped base pairs with their numbers from each other.

While the division into groups of tens makes it easy to find unit numbers, it makes it hard to define the triplets that translate to amino acids. If discussion of triplets is important, consider grouping by nines. You may also want to indicate punctuation codons.

Although there should be sufficient space between grouped pairs to separate them, if there is too much space, the continuity between them is lost.

WASTED SPACE

```
CTGCAGGCTCAAAAATGACCAGGCTAACTA
GACGTCCGAGTTTTTACTGGTCCGATTGAT
```

```
CTCGCTCAACACAGATGACCCGCTCATCTT
GAGCTAGTTGTGTCTACTGGGCCGGTAGAA
```

Here too much space is left between the lines. This results in a greater reduction of the figure, making it harder to see.

```
CAAGTCCACCCTGGACACTGATTACCAGAT
GTTCAGGTGGGACCTGTGACTAATGGTCTA
```

```
GACCAAACGGGACATGGGCTTTACTGAAGA
CTGGTTTGCCCTGTACCCGAAATGACTTCT
```

```
GGAGTTTAAAAGGCTGGTGAGTGG
CCTCAAATTTTCCGACCACTCACC
```

Compare the spacing of these two figures showing a translation into amino acids of the same strand of DNA.

RUN TOGETHER	SPACED

```
 1  CysArgLeuLysAsnAspGlnAlaAsnTyr          Cys Arg Leu Lys Asn Asp Gln Ala Asn Tyr
    CTGCAGGCTCAAAAATGACCAGGCTAACTAC        C TGC AGG CTC AAA AAT GAC CAG GCT AAC TAC  31
```

```
32  SerLeuAsnThrAspAspProLeuIlePhe           Ser Leu Asn Thr Asp Asp Pro Leu Ile Phe
    TCGCTCAACACAGATGACCCGCTCATCTTC           TCG CTC AAC ACA GAT GAC CCG CTC ATC TTC  61
```

```
62  LysSerThrLeuAspThrAspTyrGlnMet           Lys Ser Thr Leu Asp Thr Asp Tyr Gln Met
    AAGTCCACCCTGGACACTGATTACCAGATG           AAG TCC ACC CTG GAC ACT GAT TAC CAG ATG  91
```

```
92  ThrLysArgAspMetGlyPheThrGluGlu           Thr Lys Arg Asp Met Gly Phe Thr Glu Glu 121
    ACCAAACGGGACATGGGCTTTACTGAAGAG           ACC AAA CGG GAC ATG GGC TTT ACT GAA GAG
```

```
122 PheLysArgLeuBalSer                       Glu Phe Lys Arg Leu Bal Ser             144
    TTTAAAGGCTGGTGAGTGG                       GAG TTT AAA AGG CTG GTG AGT GG
```

Correspondence between triplets and the separate amino acids in the spaced version is easier to see. Note that the numbering of nucleotide bases is beside each row. While this makes a more vertically compact figure, it is harder to locate items numbered in this way. In the spaced figure, numbers are on the right. This is not commonly done but is a way to de-emphasize the numbers.

Analysis of the sequence is often the purpose of the figure. Ways of showing analysis are indicated opposite.

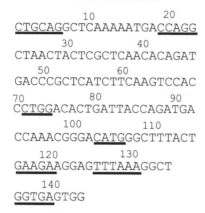

UNDERLINE

```
         10        20
CTGCAGGCTCAAAAATGACCAGG
         30        40
CTAACTACTCGCTCAACACAGAT
         50        60
GACCCGCTCATCTTCAAGTCCAC
70       80        90
CCTGGACACTGATTACCAGATGA
         100       110
CCAAACGGGACATGGGCTTTACT
         120       130
GAAGAAGGAGTTTAAAGGCT
         140
GGTGAGTGG
```

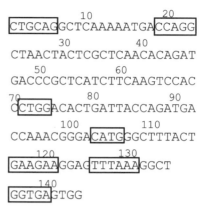

BOX

```
         10        20
CTGCAGGCTCAAAAATGACCAGG
         30        40
CTAACTACTCGCTCAACACAGAT
         50        60
GACCCGCTCATCTTCAAGTCCAC
70       80        90
CCTGGACACTGATTACCAGATGA
         100       110
CCAAACGGGACATGGGCTTTACT
         120       130
GAAGAAGGAGTTTAAAGGCT
         140
GGTGAGTGG
```

Repeats of nucleotides, regions of sequences and sites of enzyme cleavage are some aspects of sequence analysis. Above, enzyme cleavage sites are indicated in different ways. Underlining is the simplest and clearest. Boxing groups of letters is effective, but because the letters are so close together the boxes may distort or obscure the letters themselves.

Sometimes it is necessary to make several distinctions in analysis. In this case, there are other graphical possibilities.

OVERLINING, UNDERLINING, AND LINE STYLES

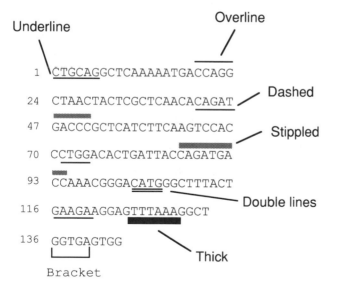

Selection of areas of a sequence is shown in various ways here. Overlining is distinguishable from underlining. Dashed lines are the least conspicuous. Stippled bars and double lines tend to fuse when reduced. Thin or thick lines are easy to distinguish, and brackets show groupings clearly.

SHADING, ARROWS, AND ASTERISKS

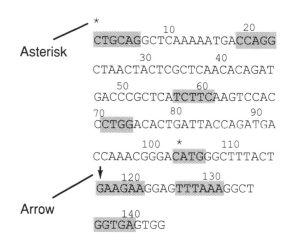

Shading areas is not a good idea because the shading obscures the letters to be emphasized. In reduction, the dots of the shading tend to fuse together and become solid black.

Make arrows and asterisks large enough to be seen and easily distinguished.

If the program for generating sequences does not have any graphic options, consider adding options to the program which would make it possible to point to areas in ways that are noticeably different.   Also, it is possible to transfer the data of the sequence to a drawing program and make additions in that program. Another choice, perhaps a simpler one, is to make the additions by hand.

Alignment of regions of sequences to show similarities or differences is shown here by using dashes to indicate gaps, upper case letters to indicate exact matches, and lower case letters to indicate no match.

SEQUENCE ALIGNMENT

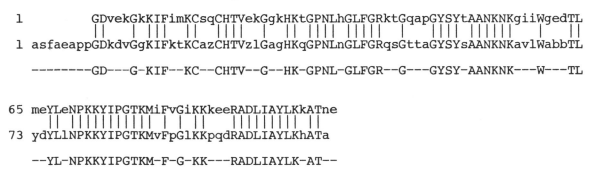

Shown above is a sequence alignment of human and parsnip cytochrome amino acids. Here amino acids are represented by single letters rather than a three letter abbreviation. The alignment is shown as it appears on the computer screen. Capital letters joined by vertical dashes denote exact alignment. The horizontal dashes in the bottom line denote gaps in alignment.

To make this figure readable and more informative, it should be rearranged and fully labeled.

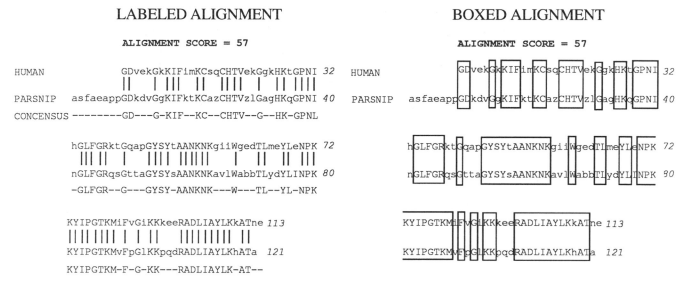

LABELED ALIGNMENT

ALIGNMENT SCORE = 57

```
HUMAN        GDvekGkKIFimKCsqCHTVekGgkHKtGPNI 32
             ||   |  |||  ||  ||||  |  ||  ||||
PARSNIP   asfaeappGDkdvGgKIFktKCazCHTVzlGagHKqGPNI 40

CONCENSUS --------GD---G-KIF--KC--CHTV--G--HK-GPNL


          hGLFGRktGqapGYSYtAANKNKgiiWgedTLmeYLeNPK 72
          ||| ||   |   |||| ||||||    |   ||  ||  |||
          nGLFGRqsGttaGYSYsAANKNKavlWabbTLydYLINPK 80

          -GLF'GR--G---GYSY-AANKNK---W---TL--YL-NPK


          KYIPGTKMiFvGiKKkeeRADLIAYLKkATne 113
          ||||||| | | ||   ||||||||||  ||
          KYIPGTKMvFpGlKKpqdRADLIAYLKhATa 121

          KYIPGTKM-F-G-KK---RADLIAYLK-AT--
```

BOXED ALIGNMENT

ALIGNMENT SCORE = 57

```
HUMAN     GDvekGkKIFimKCsqCHTVekGgkHKtGPNI 32

PARSNIP   asfaeappGDkdvGgKIFktKCazCHTVzlGagHKqGPNI 40


          hGLFGRktGqapGYSYtAANKNKgiiWgedTLmeYLeNPK 72

          nGLFGRqsGttaGYSYsAANKNKavlWabbTLydYLINPK 90


          KYIPGTKMiFvGiKKkeeRADLIAYLKkATne 113

          KYIPGTKMvFpGlKKpqdRADLIAYLKhATa 121
```

Both new arrangements will fit into one column of a journal, or are a suitable format for a slide. In the figure on the left, the three rows are labeled and the consensus score is given in the title. On the right, alignment is indicated by boxing. This eliminates the need for a consensus line and also makes the areas of homology visually clearer.

Although the use of sequences as figures is relatively new, there are some guidelines that will make them more intelligible and effective for communicating information.

Be clear about the purpose when preparing sequences for publication, slides or posters.

- To introduce a new sequence and translation, the entire sequence must be shown.

- For comparison of sequences, it might be more effective to show only the regions of greatest interest.

- To support other findings, use only what is pertinent to the finding.

Design the sequence for the medium.

- A slide of a long sequence will be meaningless to most viewers. Select only parts of a sequence for a slide. Make the labels complete and large and include a title.

- Short sequences are also better for posters, and for this purpose it is especially important that labels be large.

- While more information can be included in a sequence for publication, it will be trying and tedious for the reader to wade through a page of sequences and legends to find the points of interest. When possible, select sections that focus on the points you want to make.

- Use an appropriate format. A horizontally aligned sequence is better for a slide than one which is vertically aligned. For publication, a sequence can be planned for long and narrow column width size, or it can stretch across the width of a page, covering a whole or part of the page.

Do you really need to show the sequence?

- Can the point of interest of a sequence be stated in a sentence or two?

- Will a map or model emphasize the point as well or better than a sequence?

- Remember that the data of the sequence can be deposited in a national data base so that it is available to others.

Use graphical elements carefully.

- Be sure that elements are distinguishable from one another.

- Be sure that elements such as arrows or asterisks are large enough to be seen.

- Be sure the devices used to clarify do not obscure or distort.

Restriction Maps

Restriction maps show the sites of restriction enzyme cleavage. They may also show the lengths of the fragments. They are helpful in determining the structure of genes and in describing cloned fragments.

SEQUENCE SHOWING RESTRICTION SITES

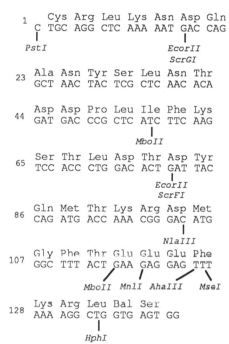

Using the same DNA strand as in previous examples, the sites of enzymatic cleavage and enzyme names are added. This works well for a small sequence. For longer sequences and for a more diagrammatic approach, a scaled map works better.

Here, the information in the sequence shown above is mapped linearly.

MAP SHOWING RESTRICTION SITES

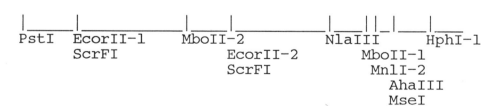

This figure shows the restriction map as it comes from the computer. The sequence is represented by the horizontal line. The enzymes are labeled, and the cleavage sites are indicated by the vertical lines.

In the restriction map just shown, the sequence line is not continuous; the enzymes actually cut the line. While this may be symbolically accurate, the sequence line is diminished in importance. There is a general impression of frequency and relative position of the enzymes, but the location of the restriction site can only be approximated. The map may be labeled more clearly and fully by transferring it to a graphic program or drawing it by hand.

REDRAWN MAP

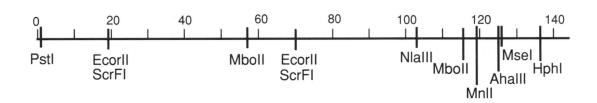

The same information is redrawn with a flexible graphic program. This diagram shows the overlapping sites more clearly and has a numbered scale to relate the total length to the restriction sites.

Restriction maps are often combined with other elements such as the sequence of a particular restricting enzyme or repeated patterns or motifs as is shown below.

ADDED MOTIFS

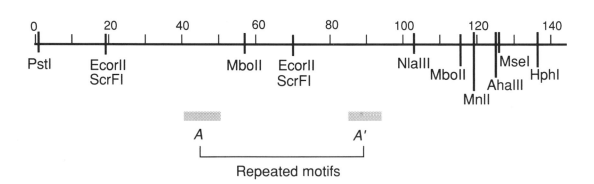

A' is a repeat of the motif, A. Both are positioned under the area in the sequence line in which they appear. Since the repeat is of secondary importance in this figure, the motif areas are indicated by stippled bars which are less obtrusive than solid lines, and also symbolize areas. Labels are the same size as the enzyme labels, but italicized to make them different.

When displaying different kinds of information in the same figure, make sure the differences are apparent visually. This can be done by spatial separation and differences in graphical devices used such as textures, weights of line, and differences in label size and style.

Circular Maps

Maps may also be shown in circular form. Plasmids, for instance, are small circular segments of DNA, and are best shown this way.

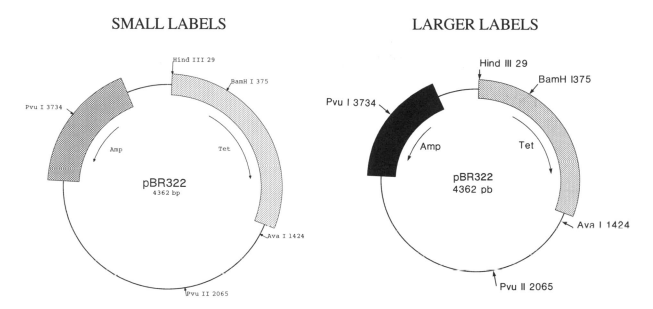

On the left is a plasmid map which shows sites for enzymatic cleavage. Regions of interest are demarcated by the hatched and cross-hatched areas. Both of these patterns are too fine-lined and close together to show up well in reduction. Labels are hard to read. On the right, enzyme labels and arrows were enlarged and "Amp" texture was darkened to distinguish it from "Tet". New and larger labels, arrows, and darkened texture for this figure were done by hand.

Mapping is a compact way to communicate large amounts of information, and is frequently used. The guidelines for effective sequences could also be used for maps.

> • Make the labels large enough to be read easily.

> • Design the map as much as possible to conform to the medium used.

> • Make use of graphic tools, such as thick and thin lines, arrows, brackets, and shading.

Molecular Models

Models are two or three dimensional diagrams of molecular structure. They are useful for study and analysis of molecules and for visualizing their spatial arrangement and interaction with other molecules. Many complex models are computer-generated using data derived from sequencing and mapping. However, artists are also extensively involved in model design, and are still coming up with new ways to display molecules. Artists continue to use the tools at their disposal to do this. The standard tools include not only pen and brush but also computers.

While some models are generated from sequences, other models of molecular structure are discovered through X-ray crystallography. The structure of a molecule may reveal function. It may reveal how it interacts with other molecules. While the shapes of molecules are hypothetical, they nevertheless allow us to model what is going on at a molecular level. The understanding of molecular structure relies heavily on pictorial presentation.

One of the simplest, and yet the most crucial, models derived from the sequence is the pattern of folding. Folding is the basis for understanding the structure of the molecule.

SEQUENCE FOLDING

The example on the left, A, is an mRNA sequence from ape beta-globulin . It shows one stem and hairpin loop fold. Here recognition and pattern of the bases is subsidiary to the folded shape. In some molecules there are many folds, so that the numbering of the folds becomes important for description. The number "1" labeling the fold is too small and hard to find (arrow). In B, the loop number is larger and positioned beside the loop. Hydrogen bonds which stabilize the folding are differentiated from covalent bonds by dotted lines.

Folding of protein is shown in the figure below.

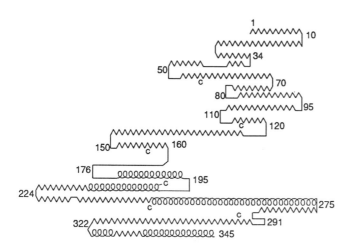

Folding of protein was predicted by the sequence method. Amino acid abbreviations are not shown here and emphasis is on the beta sheets (sharp peaks) and alpha helices (loops).

Folding diagrams are limited to one plane, but the bonding and the rudimentary probability of the structure are shown. For an idea of tertiary structure, it is necessary to simulate a third dimension.

The ribbon diagram below is one way to show three dimensional folding in a protein, based on bonding, alpha helical structure, and beta strand structure.

RIBBON MODEL

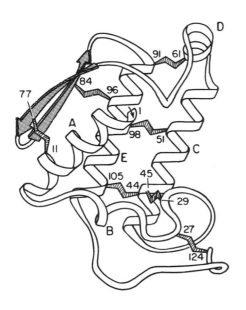

This is a schematic representation of the enzyme, phospholipase A_2. Five alpha helices (corkscrew shapes) are labeled alphabetically. Two beta strands are represented by grey arrows. Disulfide bonds are jagged, hatched shapes. The ribbons represent the sequences and the numbers show where on the sequence the bonding occurs. Depth is achieved by showing the ribbon as curving, tapering, or positioned in front or in back.

More conventional models show the bonding of atoms to form a molecule. These models are specified as skeletal, ball and stick, and space-filling. There is a great deal of symbolism involved in the representation of these models: a circle for an atom and a stick for a bond, for instance. Most of this symbolism is commonly understood and care should be taken to use it accurately, or to carefully explain any deviations from common usage. Symbolism such as size differences and tapering lines are used to convey a sense of three dimensions.

SKELETAL MODEL

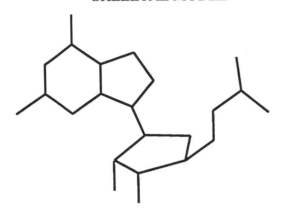

A skeletal model is the simplest model. Only the bonds with their junctions and endings are shown. An attempt is made to position them in space by angling the bonds away from a plane and slanting the plane of the pentagon.

BALL-AND-STICK-MODEL

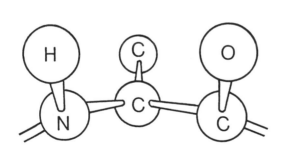

Here the ball represents the atom, the stick represents the bond. Depth in space is suggested by the tapering of the stick as well as by the stick's position in front or behind the atom. The size of the atom is also relative to its position in space. The three kinds of molecules are distinguished by labels, but for a slide, the atoms could easily be color-keyed.

SPACE-FILLING MODEL

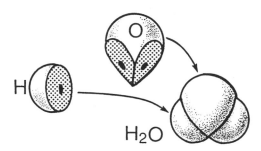

The space-filling model is more realistic than the skeletal or ball-and-stick-models, since it shows clusters of atoms adhering closely. The bonds, which are mental constructs anyway, must be imagined. The diagram here shows how the shapes of the atoms fit together to form a molecule. A three-dimensional effect is achieved by shading.

All three of these models have shortcomings, since most molecules have many more components than have been shown in the above diagrams.

Model Shortcomings

- Inside atoms are hidden by outside atoms.

- It is difficult to distinguish the different components of a large molecule.

- It is impossible to see all aspects of a molecule's structure in a two dimensional diagram.

The Computer Graphics Laboratory at the University of California in San Francisco, headed by Robert Langridge, has pioneered work in molecular modeling. This group has made great strides in overcoming the limitations of conventional models.

They have designed computer programs which show a **build up of the layers of atoms** which comprise the space filling model.

Bonds and clusters of adjoining molecules are easily **distinguished by color** in programs that they have designed.

All aspects of a molecule may be seen using a program that has been designed to **rotate the molecule**.

Other striking capabilities offered in their programs are:

- Stereoscopic presentation of molecules showing lifelike depth and dimension.

- Pocket sites for enzyme interaction, clearly color coded, and the interaction itself between two molecules.

- Movement of proteins, with possible places for fit to other molecules.

The Computer Graphics Laboratory is connected to networks all over the world and is available for consultation. They like to put their program in the users' hands and will help to customize the program.

This advanced technology offers tools to facilitate communication. However, some of these tools have outpaced the pedestrian media that are still being used: the journal, poster, and slide media. There may come a day when video tapes will be mailed instead of journals, when movies and videotapes will be used instead of slides and posters.

Meanwhile, there are still crucial decisions to make:

- What view of a three dimensional structure should be used in a two dimensional presentation?

- What will work best for the media available?

- How important is color to the presentation?

- How much money can be allotted for a given figure?

The **facet of the model** chosen for presentation should conform to the facts to be emphasized. For showing the three dimensional structure, short of using a revolving model on the computer or TV screen, several sides of the model can be depicted in several different diagrams.

For any **medium** used, a photograph of the model generated on the computer screen may be appropriate. A color slide, or an enlarged color print shot from the screen can be effective. A slide made from the computer screen, with its black background and vivid colors, can be spectacular. While the colors for a poster print lose some brilliance, the resulting figure is still striking. For publication, the negative or print must go through another step in reproduction, with a probable loss in brilliance.

Color and Cost

Often a model must be shown in **color** in order to communicate information clearly. For this reason, journals are printing more color figures taken from the computer screen. Indeed, they frequently provide an eye-catching journal cover. Color figures of this kind cannot be reproduced well in black and white. Meaning and distinctions are lost in the subtle greys that result.

The disadvantage of color prints for publication is their **cost**. While slides and prints of this kind are not unreasonable, because of the process of making a color print, the journal charge for color prints is quite high. If color is necessary to make clear distinctions, high cost may not be a deterrent. For work which is substantial in its findings, and in the labor required for the result, the high cost may be justified.

If the findings require many figures, or if grants are not large, consider using a black and white graphics program, or use an artist.

It takes time and thought to solve the problems of visual communication that continue to arise as new information is brought to light and new graphical tools are developed. However, as long as the desire to communicate coexists with a knowledge of principles of good visual communication, time and thought on this subject will be well spent.

> Most computer programs are designed for analysis, not for good graphic communication. With the help of a computer programmer, you can change a computer program to fit your needs. Or you can ask for a program that has graphical possibilities.

7

KINDS OF GRAPHS

In research, graphs of data are the most widely used means of communication. A graph turns numbers into pictures. Data evolve into bars, curves, or points which vividly show rise and fall, divergences, relationships, trends, and changes. A graph is a powerful way to show the results of a mathematical calculation.

Historically, this powerful tool of science is a recent invention, a product of the scientific revolution of the seventeenth century. It began with René Descartes' *La Géométrie,* published in 1679, in which he arithmetized geometry by fixing the positions of points on a plane by the use of coordinate axes lines.

The concept of showing change and processes by graphing also dates back to the seventeenth century, and has undoubtedly played a crucial part in the development and understanding of science. Issac Newton was the first to understand that change could be expressed graphically, although he fell back on geometrical forms in his *Principia* (possibly one reason it is so difficult to read). To describe changes, relationships, and trends in words alone is a lengthy and complicated task, and, once done, may still be hard to understand.

If you have a choice of presenting your information in tables or graphs, choose the graph. A graph conveys the information more quickly and easily than a table. It also shows the information more impressively and memorably.

On the other hand, if the information can be said in one or two sentences, or if the absolute numerical values are necessary in the presentation, use words or tables. To emphasize essential numerical data, use a graph WITH the table.

A graph is a system of connections expressed by means of commonly accepted symbols. As such, the symbols and symbolic forms used in making graphs are significant. This symbolism must be acknowledged in order to communicate clearly.

There are several commonly used graph forms, each of which shows data differently. The following pages discuss the kinds of graphs available and describe their symbolic function.

The Pie Graph

The symbol of the circle or the "pie" with its wedge-shaped pieces is satisfying and easily understood by the viewer. It shows the whole with its parts.

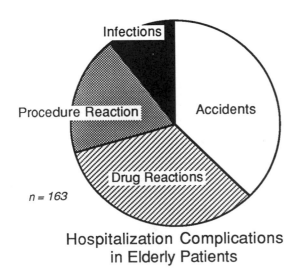

Hospitalization Complications in Elderly Patients

This pie graph shows a division of percentages. To be effective the number of divisions should be limited and the labels should be succinct. It is difficult to show and label many small divisions or percentages effectively.

The Bar Graph

The symbolism of the bar graph is as familiar to us as the yardstick or the column of mercury in the thermometer. It shows measured amounts. The simplest bar graph compares one or more sets of measurements against a single axis.

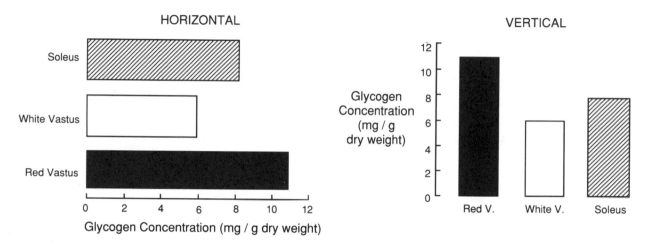

Both graphs show the same measurements of glycogen concentration in 3 different muscles taken at the same time. Arrangement may be horizontal or vertical. (Data for this and following graphs were adapted from Terjung RL, Baldwin KM, Winder WW, Holloszy JO. Glycogen repletion in different types of muscle and in liver after exhausting exercise. Am J Physiol 226: 1388, 1974.)

Horizontally arranged bar graphs are more commonly used in business than in science, but it is clearly a practical way to write long labels horizontally and without abbreviations. In vertically arranged bar graphs, however, changes have a more dramatic symbolism. "Up" is the usual symbolism for increase; the meaning of "right" is less clear. (Computer programs for graphs may call the vertical arrangement a "column graph" and the horizontal arrangement a "bar graph".) Sometimes space considerations determine whether a horizontal or vertical graph should be used.

In bar graphs, measurements made at different times may be shown. However, such measurements are static or unchanging. Separate measurements by themselves or compared to other separate measurements are essential to a bar graph.

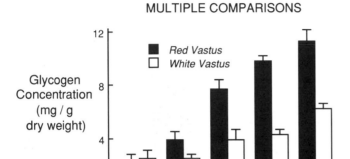

The bar graph to the left compares two sets of data measured at five different times. The red and white vastus are distinguished by shading and labeled in the key. There is no horizontal axis line because there is no second scale.

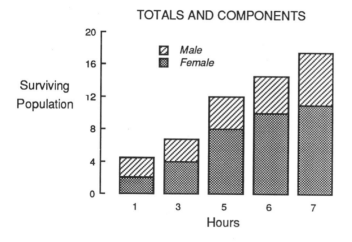

In the stacked bar graph, total measurements are compared and subdivisions of the total are also shown. This is useful when totals are more significant than components.

The Histogram

A histogram measures frequency of occurrence. It could be expressed as a series of bars, but usually shows only the tops of the bars.

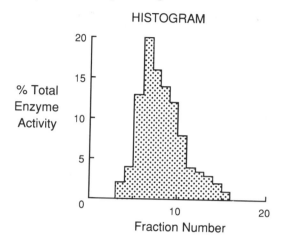

The graph on the left shows only the tops of the bars. It shows an equilibrium density distribution pattern and is a true histogram. The width of each bar represents a range of values. The shading is optional but emphasizes the area from baseline to the tops of the bars.

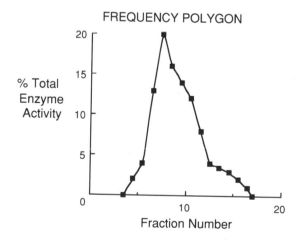

This is the same graph as above, but the frequency is plotted at the midpoint of the bars and joined by interpolated lines. This is referred to as a frequency polygon. The emphasis here is on the flow of change .

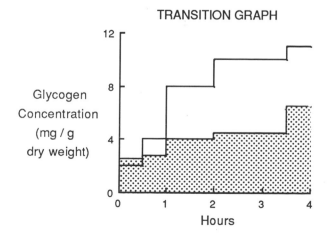

Although this graph may look like a histogram, it is actually a cross between a bar graph and a line graph. The data from the bar graph are plotted on a time scale in a series of bars showing only the tops of the bars. The area from baseline to the tops of the bars is emphasized.

The Line Graph

Decartes' fixing of a point's position on a plane by use of coordinate axes lines was naturally extended by Newton to express movement. Change is shown when the points are connected by lines. The points and lines move the eye and, like the towns and highways symbolized on a map, they simplify and clarify large amounts of information.

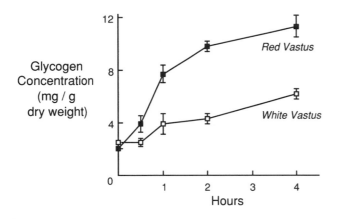

The points here represent the means of a quantity of collected data; the standard error lines show the spread. The lines joining the points create the impression of movement showing the change, trend, or comparison.

The Scattergram

The scattergram shows the influence of one variable on another. It shows the functional relationship of the variables. Points that are grouped together indicate strong correlation while points that are widely scattered indicate a weak relationship.

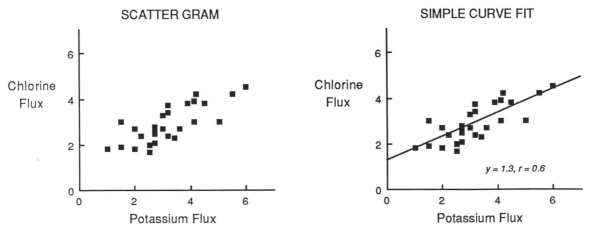

The scattergram on the left shows the relationship between chlorine and potassium flux. By adding the simple curve fit, as on the right, the correlation, or lack of correlation, becomes clearer. A computer program can be used to calculate the correlation coefficient, r.

Overlapping Graph Forms

Sometimes the information may fit several graph forms. Knowing the distinctions between the kinds of graphs and being clear about what should be emphasized will help in deciding which form of graph will work best.

PIE GRAPH OR BAR GRAPH?

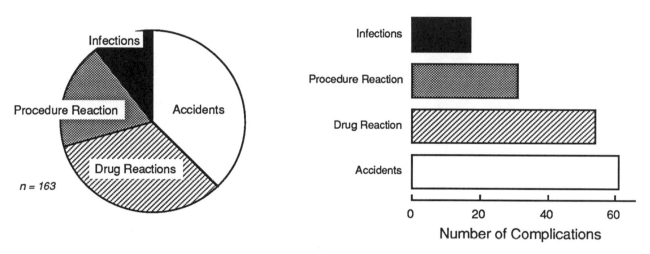

Notice how different the emphasis is in the above graphs. The total amount with its divisions is stressed in the pie graph while quantitative comparisons of the divisions are clearer in the bar graph.

BAR GRAPH OR LINE GRAPH?

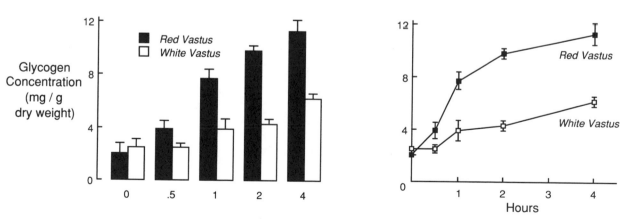

In the bar graph the difference between the red and white vastus at each time measurement is emphasized. In the line graph the change over time is more important. In the line graph, the initially lower glycogen level of the red vastus is almost obscured.

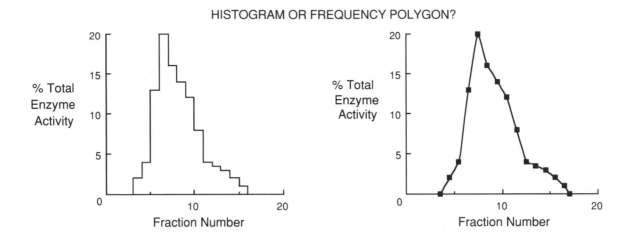

In the histogram on the left, change is expressed in a stair-like configuration.   In the polygon on the right, the same information is expressed by points and interpolated lines. In the histogram, discrete, independent but related processes are shown, while in the polygon, a dynamic process of change is emphasized.

Each graph form presents information in a special way and uses particular symbolism to communicate an appropriate message. Know what you want to say and make sure the kind of graph you select fits your message.

However, choosing the suitable graph form is only the beginning of the choices you have. The next chapter discusses the fine points of tailoring a graph that communicates your information forcefully.

8

GRAPH DESIGN

The previous chapter discussed kinds of graphs and their appropriate use. However, once you have plotted your graph in the appropriate form on graph paper or on the computer, it will still require refinement to turn it into a graph which communicates clearly and effectively.

Since graphs are symbolic representations of data, the symbolism must be understood and used correctly. There are often choices of ways to use the symbolism and while the differences are subtle, the right choice may make the information clearer. This chapter shows examples of problems of confusion and ambiguity encountered in graphs and suggests solutions.

The poor graph below, along with other graphs, is used in the following pages to illustrate common problems with axes, labels, and symbolism.

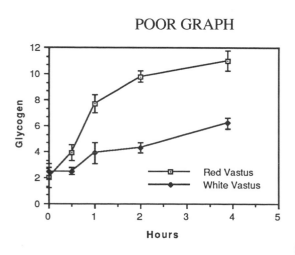

POOR GRAPH

This graph shows how long it takes to replenish glycogen in two kinds of muscle after exhausting exercise. This is shown appropriately as a time/line graph and the information is accurate. Yet this is a poor graph mainly because of axis length, tick intervals, and label size, style and position.

Axes Lines

An axis is the ruler that establishes regular intervals for measuring information. Since it is such a widely accepted convention, it is often taken for granted and its importance overlooked. Axes may emphasize, diminish, distort, simplify, or clutter the information. They must be used carefully and accurately.

The x-axis (horizontal axis, or abscissa), runs from left to right. The y-axis (vertical axis, or ordinate) runs from bottom to top.

Axes Length

To avoid wasting space, an axis should extend only to the labeled unit or minor tick closest to the last data point.

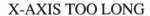

X-AXIS TOO LONG   COMPACT X-AXIS

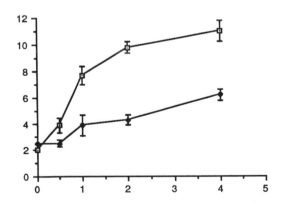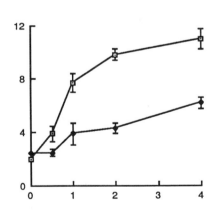

By ending the x-axis at the last data point (4 hours), the graph is more compact. In saving space, reduction in a journal is less and enlargement in a slide is greater.

Single Axis

In a bar graph, only one variable is presented. The second line is a base line which does not express anything. Below a bar graph is shown with and without the second line.

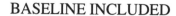

BASELINE INCLUDED   WITHOUT BASELINE

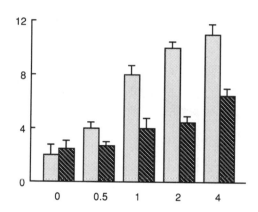
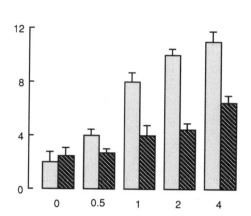

A bar graph, such as the one on the left, often shows two axes. Since only the y-axis presents data, and since the measurements on the x-axis are not regular, the horizontal baseline should be left out. This is shown in the graph on the right. In addition to having a cleaner and more open look, the grouped measurements are more clearly shown to be separate entities which may or may not be regular.

Most computer graphic programs include the nonfunctioning axis line for bar graphs with no option for removal. This is an option that could and should be included in graphic programs. In the graph without a baseline shown above, this superfluous line was removed by whiting it out by hand.

Intersecting Axes

A line graph shows axes of coordinates. The axes are two intersecting straight lines against which the relative positions of points are determined. The axes generally intersect at zero. If the two axes do not meet at zero, this fact should be indicated in a noticeable way.

INCOMPLETE Y-AXIS   AXES INTERSECT AT ZERO

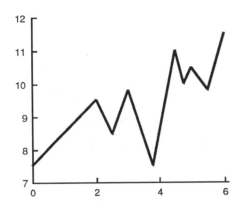   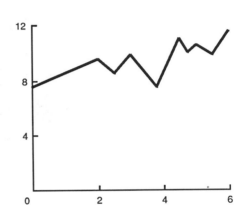

In the graph on the left, the x-axis meets the y-axis at 7. The viewer must look twice to see that the y-axis is not complete. On the right, the whole y axis is shown so that both axes meet at zero. This dramatically changes the look of the curve and while it leaves unused space at the bottom of the graph, it may give the truest picture of the data.

Starting an axis at zero may waste space at the bottom of the graph if data are limited to an area far above zero, as in the graph above. However, when comparing such a curve with others in a different y-axis range, comparisons are much clearer visually when all axes originate from zero. If changes in the curve are more important than where the curve falls on the axis, it is acceptable to start the axis at a number other than zero as long as it is clearly indicated.

Indeed, sometimes there are valid reasons for not starting an axis from zero. Certain measurements do not start at zero (pH or logarithmic scales, for example), zero is irrelevant to some scales (wavelength or absorbance, for instance), or scales start below zero. Also, information may be obscured by an axis line. But whatever the reason for not beginning an axis line on zero, it should be made visually clear that this is the case.

Two ways to show that the axes do not start at zero:

AXES OFFSET   AXIS BREAK

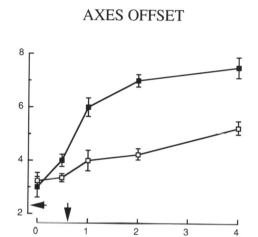
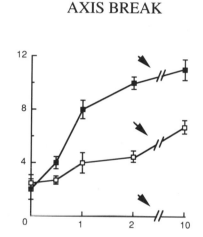

In the figure on the left, both axes have been moved aside from their original position (arrows). Not only is it obvious that the scales do not meet at zero, but this allows us to see clearly the first points with their standard errors. On the right, the time scale (x-axis) has been made more compact by the breaks indicated by the arrows. Notice that breaks are shown on the curves as well as on the axis line.

While in many computer graphic programs axes start from the first data measurement entered, there are usually mechanisms to change the axes to start from zero. Unfortunately, most programs do not offer options for showing breaks or offset axes. The graphs shown above were done in a graphing program, then transferred to a drawing program for axes changes. (See *Chapter 13, Using a Computer,* for a discussion of computer programs.)

A scale break shows an interruption of continuous units of measurements. It is not accurate to use a scale break to show unit changes.

MISUSE OF SCALE BREAK

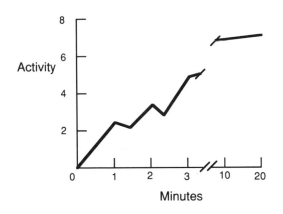

The x-axis of this graph starts out with increments of 1. After the break, it resumes with increments of 10. This is an incorrect use of the break symbol, and may be deceptive to the viewer who may not at first notice it.

If the difference in level and duration of activity after 3 minutes is not significant, it could be better said in one sentence. If the difference in level of activity after 3 minutes is important, it is adequately represented by a sampling using the same increments after as before the break. If both level and duration of activity after 3 minutes must be shown, separate the x-axis into two.

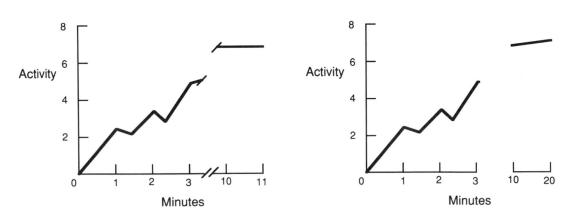

Increase in level of activity is shown on the left. Increase in both level and duration is shown on the right by dividing the x-axis into two by leaving empty space between the division. This is equivalent to making two graphs without repeating the y-axis.

Ticks

Tick marks symbolize abbreviated grid lines. To show a whole grid is not desirable since it obscures curves and causes visual clutter. The number of tick marks and labels should be as even as possible for both axes. Crowding axes with ticks and numbers clutters the graph lessening viewer comprehension. Also, one axis with crowded ticks and numbers draws attention to itself. The viewer should be able to determine easily the unit increments and minor tick division.

DIFFICULT INCREMENTS   CLEAR INCREMENTS

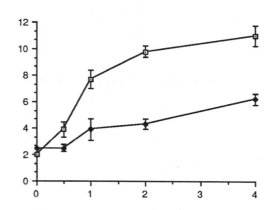 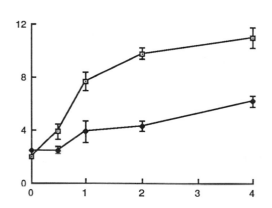

In the graph on the left, the minor ticks on the y-axis divide the units into increments of .67. This is useless to the viewer and is changed in the graph on the right. Also, since ticks measure information inside the axes lines and represent truncated grid lines, they are symbolically more appropriately shown inside the axes lines.

For ticks to be effective, it is essential that they be easily divisible.

INDIVISIBLE INCREMENTS

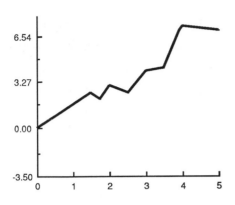

This graph has unusual increments on the y-axis which are impossible to divide without a calculator. This makes it difficult for the viewer to interpret the data.

Many graphs have odd increments because they do not start from zero, or because of the limitations of a graphing program. Try to avoid computer programs which have no option for adjusting increments.

Crowded ticks on one or both axes are commonly seen.

TICKS CROWDED ON Y-AXIS   TICKS EVEN

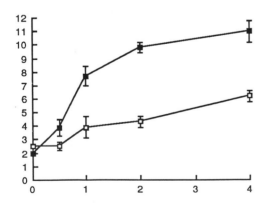
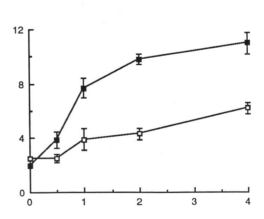

On the left the y-axis is crowded with ticks and numbers. This draws the eye away from the curves and labels and causes the viewer to wonder about the significance of the y-axis compared to the x-axis. On the right, ticks with identifying numbers are well spaced and fairly even on both axes. The ticks and numbers on this graph do not distract from the curves with their labels.

Make use of minor ticks (without numbers) to show more increments without crowding. Try to keep the maximum number of major (numbered) ticks per axis to five. More than that clutters the graph, especially since it often means using units of one or two decimals. The more digits in the number, the more crowding there will be. This is shown in the following figures.

MAJOR TICKS

MAJOR AND MINOR TICKS

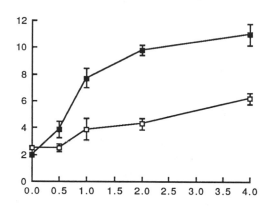
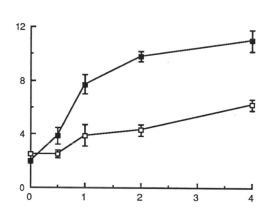

Every tick mark on the left-hand graph is numbered. Notice that the numbers are carried out to one decimal on the x-axis, causing crowding. On the right, every other tick is labeled. This is an excellent way to eliminate crowding without eliminating information.

Eliminate unnecessary zeros. This is also a cause of crowding.

EXCESS ZEROS

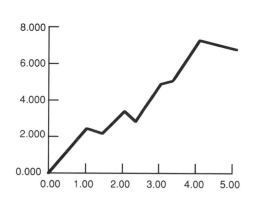

The zeros in the decimal places here serve no function and should be eliminated to avoid crowding.

An axis may be scaled in arithmetic units (linear scale) or logarithmic units (log scale). In the linear scale, as we have seen from the previous graphs, all increments are uniform and start from zero. In a log scale, units grow increasingly smaller for each cycle. For a scale of many log cycles, only the first number of the cycle need be labeled. Since the tick intervals are irregular on log scales, enough ticks should be included to show immediately that the scale is logarithmic.

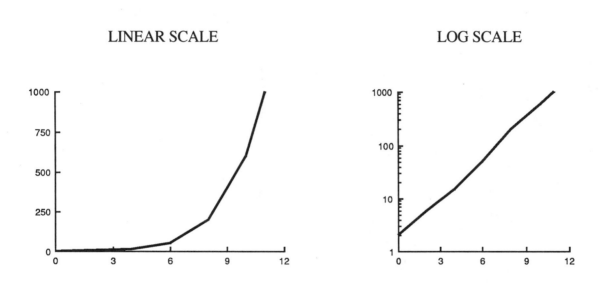

The ticks on the log scale are visual cues to the axis type. The data for both of these examples are the same. The log scale shows exponential increase and the resulting curve looks quite different from that of the linear graph. The range of data and aspects of the data which are to be emphasized will determine which scale to use.

Axes Proportions

In general, axes should not extend beyond the last data point except to end the axis with a labeled tick. Both axes should be even in length as well as number of units. However, adjustments in axes length are sometimes justified to better fit the space requirements of the medium you use, or to express the data more truthfully.

SHORTER X-AXIS   SHORTER Y-AXIS

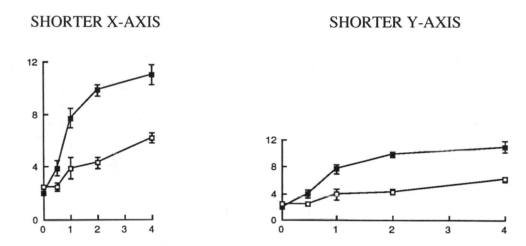

Both graphs contain the same data, but because of the change in axes proportions, the impressions from each are different. By shortening the x-axis, the curve increase is emphasized. By shortening the y-axis, the curve is flattened. Notice that the standard errors on the graph on the right make the data seem much more uniform.

By shortening the x-axis, labels may be written horizontally without increasing the reduction in a journal. If the similarity of increase of both curves is important, the shorter y-axis shows a truer picture. Also, if a wider format is desirable (for a slide for instance), a shorter y-axis works well.

Duplicate Axes

Duplicate axes are axis lines repeated at the top and right of the graph. This is referred to as "boxing in the graph" or "plot frame" in some graphing programs. These extra lines are unnecessary unless it is important to be able to make measurements across the graph. In that case, a table or grid might serve the purpose better.

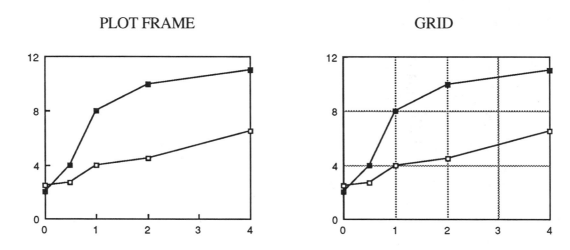

PLOT FRAME   GRID

The extra axes lines of the plot frame without ticks are not meaningful and distract from the graph curves. This is especially true with grids. Use grid lines, as on the right, only if exact measurement is most important. Be sure the grid lines are light and unobtrusive.

Computer programs make it easy to add extra lines, but they serve a dubious decorative function. Far from beautifying or compensating for paucity of information, they usually clutter or confuse.

Labels

Labels should be complete but succinct. Long and complicated labels will defeat the viewer and therefore the purpose of the graph. Treat a label as a cue to jog the memory or to complete comprehension. Shorten long labels; avoid abbreviations unless they are universally understood; avoid repetition on the same graph. A caption, for instance, should not repeat what is already in the axes labels. Be consistent in terminology.

The common problems in labeling are size, style, and placement . While labels are necessary adjuncts for identification and explanation, they should not assume primary importance in the graph. This can happen when labels are too large or too bold, or too long and complicated. On the other hand, labels must be large enough to be read easily.

In addition, label size, style, and placement may emphasize graph priorities. Variety in size and style may be functional as well as pleasing to look at, and the position of the labels may determine the sequence of attention.

Label Size

Label sizes should be in proportion to the size of the graph and to each other. While all labels must be legible, they should not dominate the graph. Number size should be smaller than axis label size, since numbers are less important. The title should be larger than the axes labels since it is a general explanation which should be read first. Subsidiary explanatory labels should be smaller than the axes labels.

Overly large or overly small labels, while an obvious problem which we all recognize, are still commonly seen.

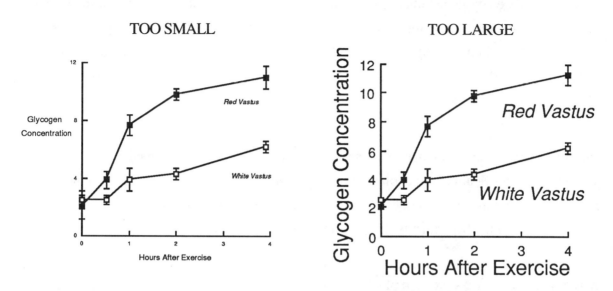

The labels on the left are hard to read; on the right, they draw too much attention. Neither satisfies us esthetically because the proportions are inappropriate. See the figure opposite, "Upper and Lower Case", for optimum size labeling.

Label Style

Upper case letters and numbers are large and more prominent than upper and lower case letters. The use of all upper case letters should be avoided for all but short labels such as a title, because they are not as easy to read as upper and lower case letters.

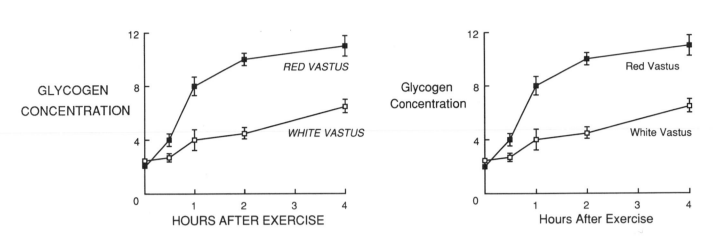

On the left, labels are all upper case. Not only is the same importance given to all labels, but the increased size of the y-axis label enlarges the total graph size. On the right, labels are upper and lower case and varied in size. This sets priorities of importance and is visually more interesting to look at.

Avoid the use of bold or thick labels except for great emphasis. Bold letters tend to dominate the graph and because they tend to become even thicker in reproduction, they are harder to read.

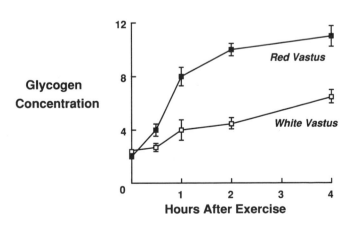

Compare the bold labeling on this graph to the plain labeling of the graphs above. Because labels are now thicker than most of the lines of the graph, they are too emphatic. The letters themselves are blurred and have lost the crispness and openness of plain labels.

Label Position

Labels may be positioned horizontally or vertically. While x-axis labels are always horizontal and centered under the axis line, y-axis labels may be either horizontal or vertical. They may be positioned to the side or above the y-axis line. Curve labels may be grouped as a legend or positioned beside each curve.

Additional labels, as for arrows or areas of interest, should be positioned with regard to symmetrical and balanced spatial arrangement. Avoid positioning labels in such a way as to cause confusion or clutter.

Take into consideration whether you will be using your graph for a slide, publication, or poster. Since horizontal labels are easier to read, for slide or poster all labels should be horizontal. For publication, the amount of reduction, the page format, and the final shape of the graph will determine whether the y-axis label be vertical or horizontal.

HORIZONTAL LABELS   VERTICAL Y-AXIS LABEL

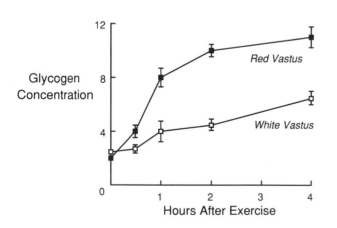
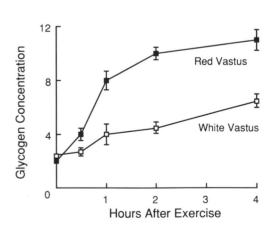

The horizontal labels on the left widen the graph. On the right, the figure is more compact. For a one-column journal, the wider figure with the horizontal labels will stretch across the page and be easily read. For reduction to one column, the squarer shape of the figure on the right will fit the column better. For slides, horizontal labels are always easier to read.

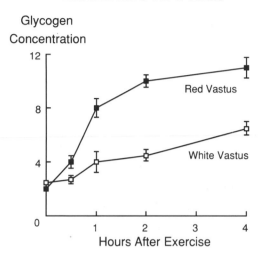

LABEL ABOVE Y-AXIS

It is not unusual to see the label positioned above the axis line. Long labels may be positioned this way to avoid aligning them vertically. For a slide with a title, however, this would not work well because the axis label and the title would be too close to each other.

Legend Labels

A legend explaining symbols used in a graph is an indirect form of labeling. For identification, the viewer must look from the curve to a legend positioned away from the curve. Identification is much quicker with direct labels positioned next to the curve. However, to avoid repetition of bar labels, or symbol labels in composite graphs, a legend can be used.

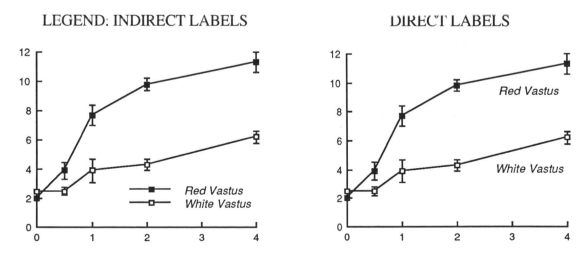

Notice how much easier it is to identify the curves that are directly labeled. In the graph with direct labels, the layout is also more pleasing. In both graphs the labels have been italicized (slanted) to set them apart from other labels.

Legends are sometimes boxed in; in some computer programs, this is automatic.

BOXED LEGEND

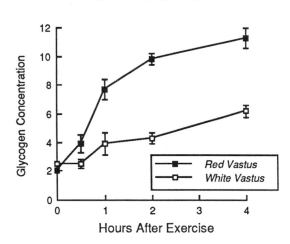

Putting a box around items serves to isolate and emphasize them. Since a legend needs no emphasis, this is not a good idea. Do not add extra lines to a graph unless you have a good, functional reason for it. The simpler and less cluttered your graph is, the better it will communicate.

Labels For Composite Graphs

When putting several graphs together to form one figure (a composite graph), several considerations are important:

- It is not necessary or desirable to repeat labels.
- Be consistent in label size, font, and style.
- Use consistent symbols.
- Design the shapes of the figures to be in conformity with each other and to fit into a format suitable for whatever medium will be used.

COMPOSITE FIGURE

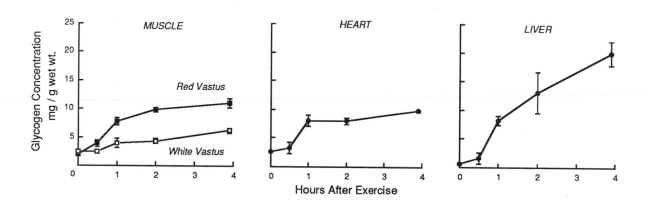

Here three graphs are shown together as one figure. The x-axes were shortened slightly to
accomodate the width of a journal page. Only one y-axis is labeled and numbered, and one label
is sufficient for all three x-axes. Each graph has a short title explaining clearly the differences
between the three. (These short titles are upper case to distinguish them from the curve labels
and italicized to set them apart from the axes labels.)

Design Symbols and Lines

Design symbols identify variables and distinguish one from the other. The most commonly used are circles, squares, and triangles, either open (unfilled) or closed (filled). Circles and triangles are more distinct than circles and squares, and open and closed symbols show distinctions most clearly.

Symbol size should be in proportion to the size of the graph and to graph priorities. In a line graph, the symbols and lines together form a picture of change or flow. Overly large symbols might distract from this picture. In a scattergram with a limited number of points, however, points might be made larger.

Avoid Xs, crosses or symbols with dots, Xs or crosses in them. In reduction they tend to fill up unevenly. Use symbols which are most distinct and use them consistently.

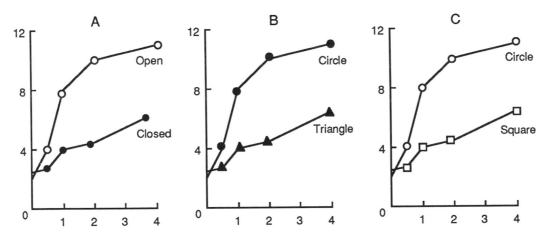

Open and closed design symbols (graph A) are the most distinct. The circle and triangle shapes (graph B) are not as distinct as open and closed symbols in graph A. The circles and squares (graph C) are least distinct, especially in reduction.

Closed symbols appear to be larger than the same size open circle (compare the open circle of graph A to the closed circle of graph B). The closed circles of graph A are slightly smaller than the open circles but the two seem the same. The square appears as largest, the circle next largest, and the triangle smallest. In graph B, the triangle is one size larger than the circle.

Lines of different thicknesses and styles can reflect priorities by emphasizing and playing down. Thick lines emphasize; thin lines play down. The solid, dashed, or dotted lines are the most easily distinguished and, of those three, the dotted line is the least emphatic, the solid line most emphatic.

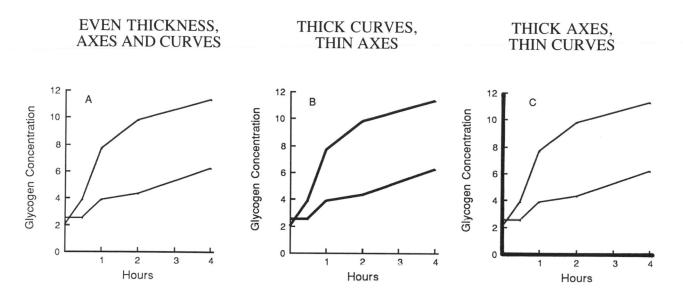

EVEN THICKNESS, AXES AND CURVES

THICK CURVES, THIN AXES

THICK AXES, THIN CURVES

In graph A, curves are visible but unemphatic. In graph B, the curves are the first thing the viewer sees. In graph C, the thick axes lines distract from labels and curves and diminish their importance.

LINE STYLES

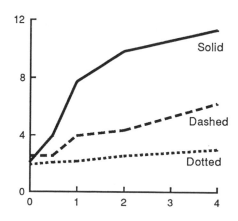

The three line styles with the most contrast are shown here. Use the dotted line for a curve with least significance. If all three curves are of equal significance and do not overlap, it is not necessary to use different line styles.

Avoid using different kinds of dashed lines in the same graph because it is difficult to tell them apart. It is not necessary and usually not desirable to vary both lines and symbols. In a series of similar graphs take care to use the symbols and lines consistently.

Texture and Contrast

Texture is a visually interesting way to clarify, emphasize and distinguish differences. Contrast, as we have already seen from open and closed symbols, accomplishes the same thing.

Stippling (small dots), hatching (lines run vertically, horizontally or diagonally) and cross-hatching are useful devices for identification and encoding. Stippling is also effective in designating areas of interest.

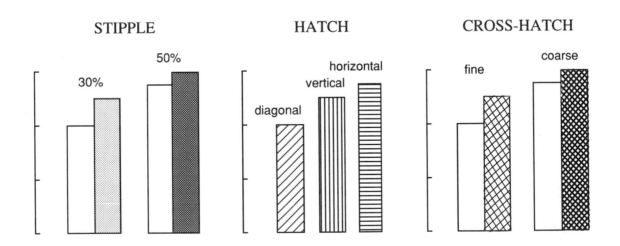

When reduced, stipples become a grey tone. Medium size dots and middle tones (30 to 50%) work best in reduction. Very fine stippling tends to drop out or become uneven in reduction. Diagonal hatching is the least ambiguous and most pleasing to the eye . Cross-hatching is darker and more emphatic. Use a fine line for cross-hatching, since thick-lined cross-hatching may fill and become black in reduction.

CONTRAST

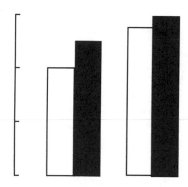

The greatest contrast is black and white. In the example on the left, the black bars are much more prominent than the white bars.

Texture should be used judiciously. Too many kinds of texture in one figure might confuse and distract from the message. Use texture and contrast as an accent or highlight to clarify and simplify as well as to attract the viewer's attention.

ARROWS AND BRACKETS

Arrows are symbols which draw the eyes' attention to an object or event or which denote motion. Arrows are not appropriate for leaders (lines) from labels to the object labeled. Plain, thin lines are best for this.

Arrows effectively indicate occurrence or direction of an event.

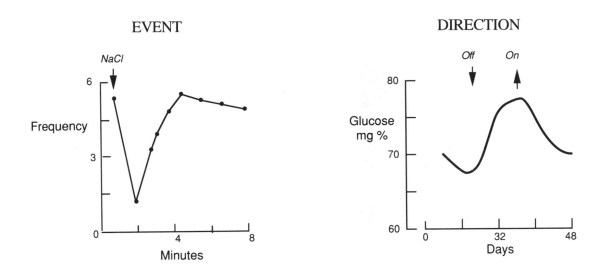

On the left, the arrow shows the time of administration of NaCl. On the right, the up and down directions of the arrows symbolize on and off.

Brackets or stippled areas are useful to indicate events which occur over a space of time.

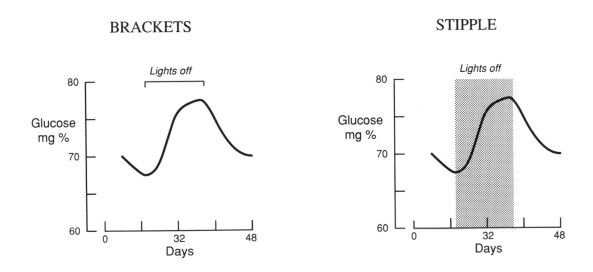

Either brackets or stipple may show an event which occurs over a space of time. The brackets on the left show clearly the duration of the event and the eye approximates the relationship of the duration to the curve changes. The stippled area on the right crosses the curve indicating exactly where the event changed the curve. However, stippling shades the curve and visually interrupts the flow of the line.

The problems discussed in this chapter have to do with clear use of symbolism, proportion, contrast, composition, and texture. These are essential components for communication of sophisticated information. While they are artists' tools, understanding of, and familiarity with their use, may be learned from observation and trial.

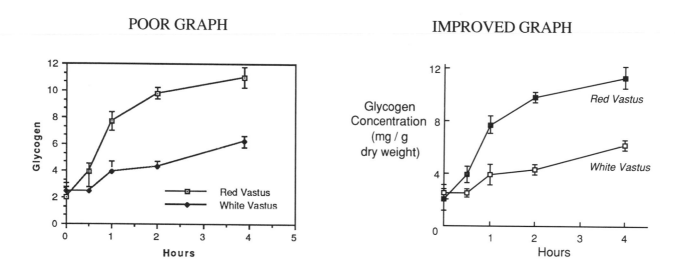

The poor graph on the left was shown at the beginning of the chapter. The improved graph on the right shows the changes in axes, labels, and symbols which result in a clear, handsome graph.

Look critically at graphs in journals, slides, and posters. Try to analyze why they are good or bad. Ask yourself how you could improve them.

9

THE JOURNAL FIGURE

Throughout the preceding chapters, differences between figures for publication and slide have been pointed out. In this chapter, the special requirements for publication in journals will be discussed. Succeeding chapters will deal with slides and posters.

Although scientists communicate in various media, from a black and white figure for a paper to a full screen, full color movie, the three most commonly used media are the published paper, the lecture and the poster presentation. Each of these three media have assets and liabilities which must be taken into account.

Just as our clothes fit the weather, graphics should fit the medium. Although it may save money and time to use the same art work for a slide, such savings are usually at the cost of good communication. A good figure fits its surroundings. The time and effort spent "dressing" a figure appropriately reflect consideration for the audience and the message.

The difference between a good published figure and a slide may be only a matter of adding a title, or it may be a whole new figure. Whatever it takes, if it gets the message across more quickly and easily, it will be worthwhile.

Publication in journals is expected from scientists and is, if not an every day occurrence, at least a yearly occurrence. Publication in books, on the other hand, is a more momentous and rare occurrence. For this reason, the following pages are specifically directed towards published figures appearing in journals. In most cases, the requirements for books are similar.

A published paper with its illustrations is the most formal and weighty method for disseminating scientific findings. Because the printed page is available for scrutiny by generations of readers, great care should be taken in the writing, and the same care should be taken with the illustrations.

For the reader, this durability and availability are **assets**. A paper may be carried around and read at the reader's convenience. The reader may spend as much or as little time on it as he/she wishes. Details may be included which the reader may study or skip.

The published figure also presents **challenges** which must be met. Chief among these are reduction and accommodation of the figure to limited space and shape. There may also be limitations on the number of figures allowed and page costs may be a consideration in some journals. Some or all of the cost of color illustrations must be borne by the author and greatly exceed conventional page charges.

The first step to producing an effective journal figure is to know the journal. Instructions to authors in the journal are the first clue.

Journal Instructions

These instructions to authors are not always easy to find, but if they are not in the front or back, look in the table of contents or in the first issue of the volume or write the editorial office. Instructions concerning figures may be a paragraph or a page. They will tell you whether to send originals or photographs; they may inform you of expected reduction and instruct you as to labeling style and size and the kinds of symbols to be used. Whether instructions be sparse or detailed, be sure to read them. Also, look through the journal, noticing such things as number of columns, style of labeling, figure reduction, and figure layout.

Reduction

The final reduction of a figure is not always predictable. It depends on journal size, format and editor. However, if you design for maximum reduction within the journal format, your figure should be legible. Maximum reduction usually means reduction to one column width of a two or three-column page ($2^3/_8$ inches to $3^1/_2$ inches; 6 cm to 9 cm). In a one-column journal, however, final reduction will depend upon the shape of the graph.

The journal may instruct you to design the figure to fit the page economically. Since wasted space costs the journal money, the object of the editor and lay-out artist is to reduce and position the figure within the surrounding text in a way that is compact not only on the page but in the context of the whole article. This may result in a final reduction to less than one-column width.

In a journal with **two columns**, a square shaped figure will usually suffer less reduction than a long, narrow figure.

ONE COLUMN WIDTH

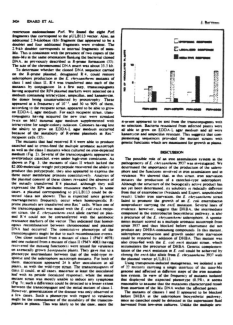

This figure is close enough to being square to occupy all of the one-column width. The letter size is about the same size as the text and is easily read. Bars are easily differentiated.

Below is a figure which has unused space around it.

LESS THAN ONE-COLUMN WIDTH   ONE-COLUMN WIDTH

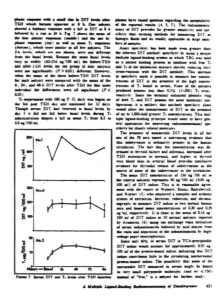

On the left, the composite figure has been reduced to less than one-column width. Notice the unused space on the sides of the figure. This reduction is reasonable since labels are legible and points and lines are easy to see. On the right, the figure has been enlarged to fill the entire column width. Notice the corresponding height of the figure,which now occupies more than half of the column.

The left-hand figure above shows how it actually appeared in the journal. In the interest of saving space, the journal reduced the figure to take up less than a column width. On such a long figure, there is room to arrange the y-axis labels horizontally for easier reading and pleasing composition.

Design your figures for the appropriate reduction.

To predict figure reduction, measure the figure dimensions. Make a box of these dimensions and draw a diagonal line from the lower left corner to the upper right corner of the box. Measure the journal column width and fit that measurement from the left hand axis to the diagonal line. Draw a vertical line from that point on the diagonal line to the lower axis. You can see how much vertical space your figure will occupy in the column.

PREDICTION OF REDUCTION

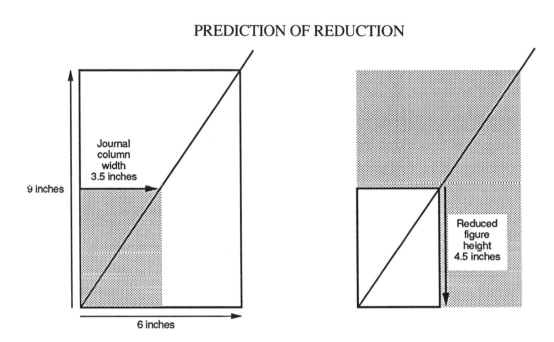

The original figure on the left measures six by nine inches including the labels. The shaded rectangle indicates the width of one column in the journal for which it is intended. On the right, the open box indicates the height of the reduced figure, derived by drawing a vertical line from the measured column width point on the diagonal line to the horizontal baseline.

If the reduced figure height occupies half or close to half of the entire column height, as this one does at 4.5 inches, it is safe to assume that it will be reduced still further to conserve space.

Avoid exaggeratedly long or wide shapes. When plotting graphs, make the axis lengths as even as possible.

Format

Design the figure for the journal. The journal format (page size and shape, and number of columns) plays a role in determining reduction. For this reason and for a figure to be maximally effective, consideration of journal format is essential in planning the shape of the figure.

One-Column Journal

The one-column journal is perhaps the most difficult to design for. The most suitable figures are those that are wider than they are long.

PAGE EXAMPLE

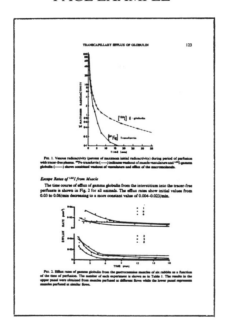

There is more wasted space around the tall top figure than the wide bottom figure. Both figures have the same reduction, but the wide bottom figure wastes less space and has more pleasing proportions on the page.

The top figure would benefit from an expanded x-axis. Both figures have room for horizontal labels on the y-axis.

An unsatisfactory alternative to wasting space with a tall figure in a one-column journal is to enlarge it to fit the column or page width. This can be seen in the following figure.

FIGURE TOO LARGE

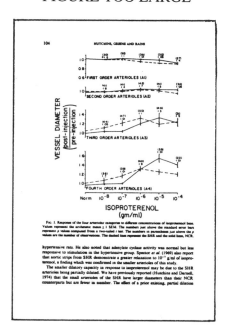

Although this figure fits the column width, it takes up most of the page. The label size is much larger than the surrounding text , giving it an exaggerated prominence. At half this size, it could still be easily read. The space between the two bottom graphs could be reduced and the y-axis label could be arranged horizontally on four lines to better fit the space.

An excellent way to save space in a one-column journal is to design side-by-side composite figures

ONE-COLUMN COMPOSITE

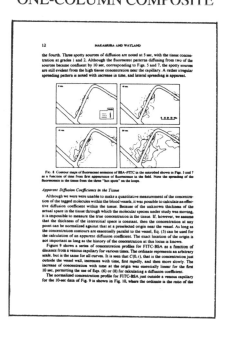

There is little wasted space in this figure since the overall shape is wider than it is tall. A wide figure has better proportions for one-column journal format and wastes less space.

It is not always possible to design wide figures or to combine figures side-by-side. But when planning figures, keep in mind journal format. Make figures conform as closely as possible to the space.

Two-Column Journal

There are more options for figure position and shape in a two-column journal. The figure may be reduced to one-column or it may stretch across the page. In rare instances, it may occupy an entire page.

ONE AND TWO TWO-COLUMN WIDTHS

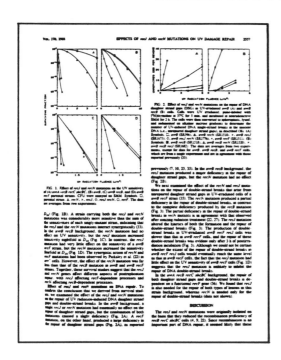
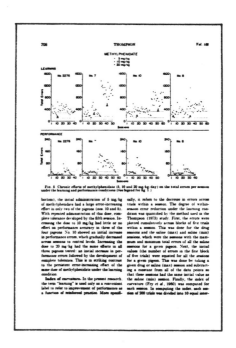

The composite figures on the left fill one-column widths. The figure on the right stretches across the page, occupying two columns and the center space between the columns.

Three-Column Journal

While two-column journals are the most common, three-column journals are becoming increasingly frequent. There are even more options for figure shape and position with three columns. In addition to occupying one, two, or three columns, a figure may spread over parts of several columns.

THREE-COLUMN PAGE

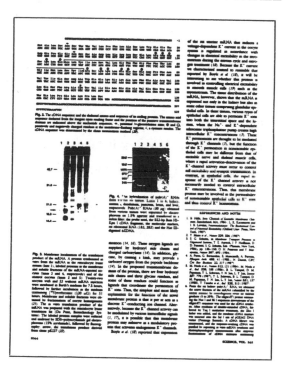
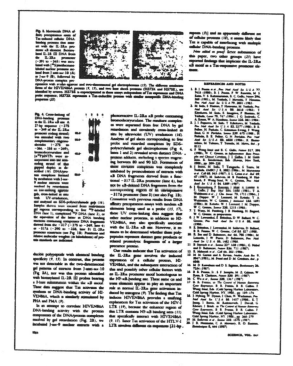

The layout on the left shows a top figure occupying two columns and, below it, two one-column figures. On the right, the top figure occupies one and a half columns with the caption wrapping around it. Below it, the gel occupies half of a column surrounded by its caption.

There are many variations in figure layout for different formats. While the researcher does not have a great deal of control over the layout, it is important to be aware of the possibilities, keeping in mind the fact that every journal aims for a compact and space-saving layout within whatever format is used.

Labels

Figure **titles** are not used in journals. The information in a title, along with a more detailed figure explanation is contained in the caption beneath the figure. The **caption** itself is an integral part of the final published figure on the page. Although occasionally a caption will be placed on the opposite page from the figure, as with a full-page photographic plate, it is generally positioned close to the figure. It may even wrap itself around the figure, as can be seen in the previous example.

Label Position

The position of the label on the x-axis is always horizontal, while for the y-axis it may be vertical or horizontal. Horizontal labels are always easier to read, but if a y-axis label is long and cannot easily be broken into several horizontal lines, it should be positioned vertically.

HORIZONTAL OR VERTICAL LABELS?

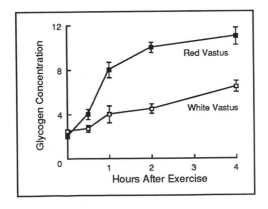 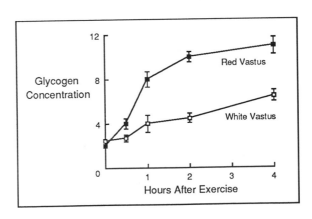

On the left, the y-axis label is vertically aligned. This maintains the almost square shape of the figure and is suitable for reduction to one column of a two-column journal. For a one-column journal, however, the horizontal alignment shown on the right is preferable because it creates a wider figure which fills a one-column space better.

Another option is to position the label above the y-axis. This is a way to maintain the ease of horizontal reading while still using space economically.

LABEL ABOVE THE Y-AXIS

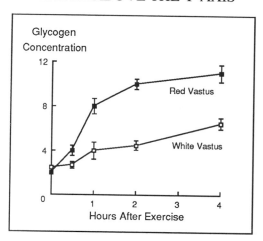

This y-axis label is divided into two lines. The square shape of the figure makes it suitable for reduction to one column while retaining the easy-to-read horizontal labels. If a label is so long that it occupies three lines above the y-axis, it would be better to position it vertically. As well as looking unwieldy, three lines of labeling will elongate the figure.

Label Style and Size

Label size in the reduced figure should not be smaller than the print on the page. Nor should it be much larger. Journal text is 8 to 10 point size, so ideally the reduced label size should not exceed 12 point. This means that if the original will be reduced by half, the labels on the original should be 24 point. Size of numbers and subsidiary labels may be smaller (18 point). For photomicrographs, labels may be larger (14 to 20 point) because of the difficulty of seeing smaller labels on such figures.

APPROPRIATE LABEL SIZE

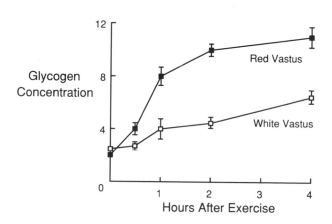

The original of this computer-drawn graph was 4.5 inches wide by 3 inches tall. It was reduced to 77% of the original to fit into a 3.5 inch one-column width. The reduced label size is 12 point for the axes labels and 10 point for all other labels.

The label style is plain for the numbers and axes, italics for the curve labels. Helvetica font is used throughout. To check for legibility of labels, reduce the figure on a photocopying machine to the required journal dimensions.

Some journals require that keys or explanatory labels be described in the caption. Others ask that there be no numbers or letters demarcating composite graphs one from the other. There are even some journals that ask that there be no labels. Check the journal instructions before labeling the figures.

Consistency

Consistency of size, shape, nomenclature, and symbols is extremely important to the smooth flow and easy understanding of information. In planning your figures, think of them in terms of the whole paper and design original figures which are uniform in size.

If figures made at different times or from various sources are used, consider adapting them to conform to a consistent style.

Final Preparation

After the figures are completed, and before any required photography, check them carefully for errors. Ask colleagues to check them for errors. Changes made after photography are costly and time-consuming.

Examine the final figure carefully for consistently black lines and clean white background. Reduce the figure on a copy machine to check label legibility and to make sure that lines do not drop out and that stippled areas do not fade.

If glossy photographs are submited, check them for good contrast and sharpness of line. In the case of continuous-tone illustrations, check the tonal range and faithfulness to the original.

If you want figures to appear near each other or with specific text, indicate this clearly on a cover sheet.

When you mail originals, put a cover sheet over them or place them in a separate envelope to keep them clean and intact. If you mail photographic prints, avoid indentations made by paper clips or ball-point pen labels on the back. When mailing, use heavy cardboard to protect figures from bending.

All figures must be numbered consecutively to conform to the text and caption. Check to make sure numbering is correct. Number lightly on the cover sheet or on the back of the figure, or number on gummed labels applied to the figure back.

The Printing Process

When the paper is typeset, blank space is left on the page into which the line figures are inserted. For each line figure, a high-quality positive print (called a photomechanical transfer print, or PMT, sometimes called a "stat") is made in the final size and this PMT is pasted into the opening. The PMT made from high-contrast or line art records only black and white. A negative of this whole page with type and PMT in place is then made and used to make the final printing plate.

Continuous tone materials (photographs) are handled differently, since they must be converted into half-tones (screened). When the page is typeset, an opening (window) is left in the size in which the final half-tone is to be printed. A negative is made of this whole page, and the half-tone negative which has been made in separate process is fitted into the window negative of the text page. Once all page negatives are completed, their images are transferred to a metal printing plate. The plates are attached to the printing press, inked, and run in the offset process.

Color

One of the reasons why color illustrations are so expensive is that the process for producing color figures is complicated and demands special care and high technology. The cost of a color plate in a journal must be borne by the author.

A separate printing plate must be made for each color. If **spot color** (one color) is used, as for specific columns in a bar graph, the artist must prepare a separate overlay for the color area. This overlay must be in exact registration with the black and white original and the desired color must be indicated. Separate negatives are made of the original and the overlay, and separate plates are made from these negatives.

For **full color** reproduction, as of a photograph or full color drawing, the original must be scanned either mechanically or digitally using filters to separate the colors. The scanning process is analogous to the half-tone process in that tiny dots are created to generate the final printed image. All of the colors of the original are created by mixing dots in various proportions of three printing colors plus black. A negative is made for each color and black; all four of these negatives must be in precise register. Often color corrections must be made modifying the negative. Four metal printing plates are then made from the four negatives, which are put on the printing press in register. When the paper moves through the press, an image from each color is impressed on the paper.

Proofs

Journals usually send proofs to the author. **Galley proofs** are made before final page make-up has been done and show text in long blocks of type. However, to save time, most journals now skip galley proofs and go directly to **page proofs**. The author sees photocopies of the final typeset pages with final size line art in place, and windows (blank spaces) where half-tones are to appear.

Half-tones, reduced as they will appear in print, are supplied on separate sheets at the end of the manuscript. The quality of proof reproduction is not as good as in the final print appearing in the journal.

At the page proof stage it is too late to change the position or size of a figure. Special requirements for figures should be indicated on the original manuscript.

> Any changes that you make which correct your own errors will be at your expense. The journal pays for errors it commits. Proof the figures and text carefully for errors.

10
SLIDES

A slide is usually seen for less than thirty seconds, so its impact has to be immediate. For this reason, figures for slides must be especially simple and succinct. A good slide makes no more than three points and these points augment, emphasize, and explain the speaker's words.

Sometimes speakers try to make one slide do the work of many. The result is visual confusion. For complicated subject matter, it is far better to use two or three simple figures than one complex and usually cluttered and unclear figure. Your audience may fall asleep while you are spending minutes trying to clear the confusion.

In addition, use of a series of slides which build on each other helps to create a dynamic and suspenseful flow of information. This can be a most effective teaching tool.

COMPLICATED SLIDE

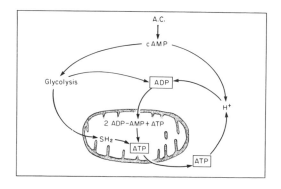

This slide will take considerable explanation and is confusing on first view. Although all the information shown here is necessary to describe the cyclical process, it could be presented more gradually and simply.

Starting simply and gradually adding information is a much more effective way to communicate. Notice that every addition increases the overall size of the figure, resulting in increased reduction.

SLIDE 1

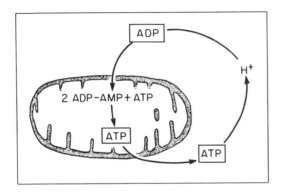

This slide shows one ATP-ADP cycle. The information here can be grasped quickly, so that the slide need not be left on for long. This and the following slide figures are shown in an appropriate slide format : a horizontally aligned rectangle.

SLIDE 2

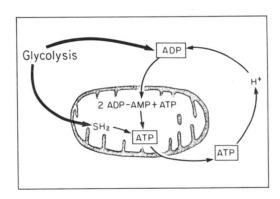

In this slide, another unit of information is added which increases the overall size of the original drawing. This results in increased reduction in the slide format. Thicker arrows and larger labels on the new information , however, clarify and emphasize the new addition.

SLIDE 3

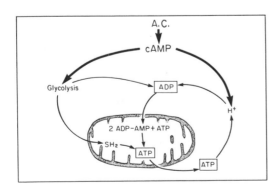

The addition of more information makes a complicated, crowded slide. However, because the viewer now has a background for the newest complicating factor, attention is focused on the new addition with its thicker lines and larger labels.

What is an overwhelming amount of information when presented at one time, can be easily assimilated when presented progressively.

Another reason for keeping slides as simple as possible is that they must be legible from the back of the auditorium. Although slides projected onto a large screen may seem gigantic from the front row, they appear much smaller in the back row. The previous complicated slide might not be legible except for the enlarged new labels.

Slide Format

The outside dimensions of slides which fit into the standard cassette are 2 by 2 inches. Within these four square inches, is a mat which determines the shape of the slide on the screen. Because they are usually made with 35 mm film, the format of the slide is controlled by this film size.

Slides have a limited number of options for format or shape. The format of the slides in the previous figure is the most common. Notice that the shape is more horizontal than it is vertical or square. This is an effective shape for slides and can be easily seen from the back row.

HORIZONTAL FORMAT

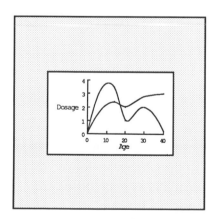

This format and the following format examples are shown actual size. A slide with a horizontal format occupies the middle of the screen. It is at eye level and is easy to read.

There can be problems with the same two by two inch slide format redrawn vertically.

VERTICAL FORMAT

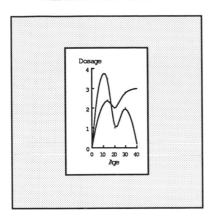

This slide format accommodates a vertical figure nicely. However, from the back row, the heads of people in front may hide the bottom part of this graph. Because a slide screen reaches to the floor does not mean that all of that space is usable.

Try to design horizontal figures for slides.

SQUARE FORMAT

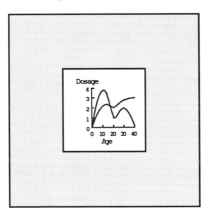

A square format results in a smaller slide which occupies less of the screen. The surrounding mat takes up more of the space. This square format is advantageous for a square figure in eliminating wasted space on the sides.

To show a square figure to larger advantage, a super slide format may work better.

SUPER SLIDE

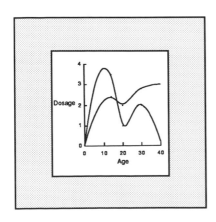

The surrounding mat of a super slide is smaller than the square format, resulting in a slide that fills more of the screen. However, the length of this format is the same as that of the vertical slide, and the bottom part of this format may not be seen easily from the back. Also 35 mm film will not fit this format.

Knowledge of the room or auditorium in which your slides will be shown is helpful in planning for vertical or super slides.

Labels For Slides

In general, effective labels for slides are briefer and larger than those for publication. Plain or thin labels are more readable and in better proportion to the rest of the figure than bold, thick letters. Bold labeling should be saved for special emphasis. All labels should be horizontal for easy reading. There are ways to arrange even long labels horizontally without excessive reduction.

Long labels may be divided into several lines and aligned horizontally; the figure may be designed to leave room for horizontal labels, or labels may be positioned at the top of the y-axis.

LONG Y-AXIS LABELS

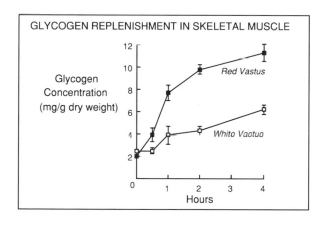

Long y-axis labels in this slide have been aligned horizontally. This is easy to read, but compare the reduction to the following slide.

DIVIDED Y-AXIS LABELS

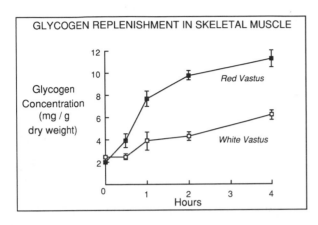

The label describing the units has been divided, so that "Concentration" is now the longest word. Compare the reduction of this figure to the one on the previous page. It is slightly less reduced.

DECREASED GRAPH WIDTH

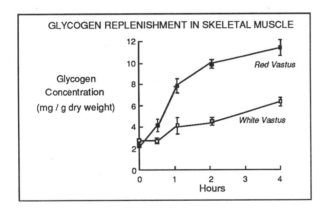

Another solution for long labels is to reduce the width of the graph itself. This leaves room for fairly long horizontal labels. The reduction is the same as in the previous graph.

LABEL ABOVE Y-AXIS

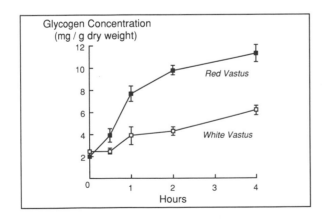

The y-axis label has been positioned above the axis line here. Even though this increases the height of the graph, the overall reduction is the same because the title has been eliminated. This kind of labeling, does not work well with a title. The shape of the figure becomes even taller, with attendant reduction, and labels look crowded and too close together.

Plan figures to accommodate horizontal labeling.

A title for a slide is a brief but informative summary of information. It should be concise and should not repeat what is contained in the axis labels.

LONG TITLE   CONCISE TITLE

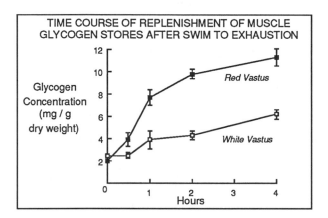

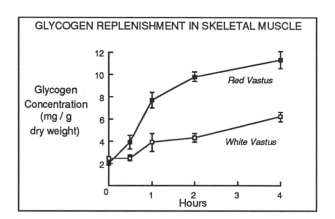

The length of the title on the left is daunting. The only new information added has probably already been described in methods. The title on the right is concise and serves as a cue or reminder.

Although a title may be an asset to a slide, it is not always necessary. The speaker's words may be enough to identify the slide. Also, series of slides which are similar except for one variable may be labeled quite briefly with only the name of the variable.

Color

A good black and white slide is classical and elegant and suffices in almost all situations. However, a color slide can charm an audience and provide variety. More than that, it can be an excellent explanatory tool. **Color keys**, used throughout a talk to denote specific entities, are an easy and pleasurable way to follow the flow of information. They can unify as well as clarify. Color in molecular models is used as a key and is often essential for clarity.

Spot color in otherwise black and white drawings is useful to accentuate or emphasize. In using color as an accent, stick to primary, bright, and clear colors for the best effect. Too many colors may be distracting and areas of color that are too small may not show up at all.

Full color, as in photomicrogaphs or full color drawings, may be essential for purposes of identification. It may be a way to capture the audience's attention. The negative of a color photomicrograph may be used as a slide with little loss of brilliance. A positive transparency must be made of a color drawing with an attendant loss of brilliance. Use of strong primary colors on a neutral, rather than white, background is effective for a slide.

Photographing color drawings for use as slides is not easy, as the photographic exposure must be exactly right to avoid an overdark or washed out projection image. A color slide which looks satisfactory on a slide viewer may project poorly. Try out each slide in a suitably sized room.

Color may be added to negative slides with dyes or color tapes. Color background slides may be made from the black and white original. In this kind of slide, the black lines of the original figure appear as white. If these lines are very thin, they are hard to see. Plan for this kind of slide by making lines thicker. Avoid using drawings with complex lines and stipple for this process since their tonality is reversed causing strange and confusing effects.

Color slides should be used with discretion, not just because they are more costly and time-consuming than black and white slides, but because they may not serve the purpose well. Color can be distracting as well as informative. Have a good reason for using color, not just availability or looks. The purpose of the slide is not to dazzle, but to inform.

Slides From Books and Journals

In the course of being printed, figures in books and journals have undergone several processes of degradation, i.e. photographs made of photographs . Even in the best quality reproduction, there is a loss of sharpness, a possible unevenness of tone, and in the case of continuous-tone figures a screening into small dots. When projected, flaws become more apparent.

Labeling suitable for a published figure is often too small to be read easily in a slide. The caption that accompanies a figure is most certainly too small to be read and much too long to be included in a slide. Also the shape of the printed figure may not fit the slide format well.

In addition, most often such a figure taken from the printed page does not completely fit the purpose. It contains more information than is needed. How often have you heard a lecturer say, "Don't pay any attention to this part of the slide"? If all the information on a slide is not valuable to the audience, leave it out. There are ways to adapt the printed figure to a slide, so do not impose this burden of translation on the audience.

With scissors, tape, white correction paint, photocopying machine, and minimal time and effort a printed figure may be transformed into an adequate slide.

JOURNAL FIGURE

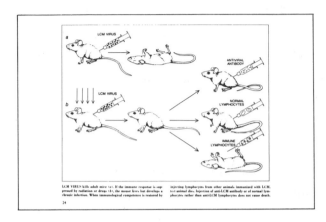

This figure from *How the immune response to a virus can cause disease* by A.L. Hotkins and H. Koprowski* is an excellent journal figure which serves the authors' purpose nicely. However, it contains too much information for one slide, the legend is illegible and unnecessary, and it does not fit the slide format well.

SLIDE FIGURE

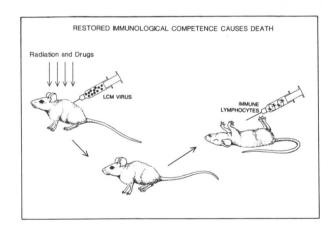

One pathway has been selected for a slide. The selected parts were cut out and glued to a white background. Additional labels, such as the title and explanation for the arrows were added. The layout was designed for minimum reduction in the slide format.

Enlargement may magnify printing flaws. Notice, also, that the photocopy machine thickens lines. This is noticeable in the labeling where parts of letters fill and blur together. However, this edited version is simpler, more succinct and effective than a straight copy of the original figure.

---

* Scientific American, January 1973, volume 228, number 1.

Overhead Transparencies

An alternative to using slides is the overhead transparency. These are figures done on transparent film and placed on an overhead projector which transfers the figure by means of lens and light to a screen, wall, or blackboard.

Some advantages of overhead transparencies are:
- They may be used in a fully lighted room.
- The speaker faces the audience, allowing better audience contact.
- Additions may be made directly on the film by marking pen or by previously prepared overlay sheets.
- They are inexpensive to make.
- They may be made quickly, especially by using the copy machine with compatible transparent plastic sheets.
- Color is an easy option using color markers, color transparent film, and transparent color tapes and press-on letters.

Overhead projectors are usually available in classrooms and lecture halls and can be effective in both small and large settings. It takes little time to learn to set up and operate the projector, so that those who have never used this method of projection could easily experiment with it. Some speakers find they are more comfortable with this direct and simple way of presenting figures.

The best overhead transparencies, like slides, have limited information and large and succinct labels. The buildup of information can be dynamic when the speaker draws directly on the transparency being projected, or adds transparent overlays.

11
POSTERS

A poster at a scientific meeting is an enlarged graphic display containing a title, the authors' names and institution, and text and figures explaining research. This form of presentation was developed as a way to handle the increased size of meetings and the growing number of presenters. Where formerly all information was conveyed in fifteen minute talks, now there is a choice of talk or poster, or posters only. This method of presentation has advantages and limitations.

Some of the **advantages** of posters are:
- They may be studied at leisure or quickly scanned.
- They offer personal contact with interested viewers.
- They may be seen as a whole entity.
- They can be more informative than a talk.
- It is a <u>visual medium</u> and excellent for illustrations.

Some of the **limitations** of posters are:
- The audience is not captive but must be attracted to the presentation.
- The viewer is not comfortably seated.
- Space is limited, so the poster must be selective.
- Text and figures must be easily seen from a distance of three to four feet.
- Posters take more time to prepare and cost more money than slides.

Plan the Poster

Planning is the most time-consuming and crucial part of the poster. The **amount of information** to be included is the primary consideration.

Unfortunately, many presenters use the poster as an enlarged journal paper.

THE JOURNAL PAPER PRESENTED AS A POSTER

The text in this poster is written as if it were for publication. Even if it were large enough to be read easily, the sheer amount is overwhelming and discouraging. None but the most determined viewer will stand for the required time to read through all of this.

Sadly, too many scientists think an "information-packed" poster conveys the impression of highly productive research. It does not. The resulting crowded and confusing presentation obscures any central ideas and conveys the message that the research may be equally unclear.

Limit your information. Get to the heart of the matter and leave out the rest. In planning what you want to say, pick out no more than three points which you think are most important and focus on them. If you can get across even one point clearly and quickly to your viewer, your poster is successful. Remember that you are there to answer questions and fill in details. If necessary, make use of printed summaries for viewers who are interested in more detailed information.

Poster Instructions

Poster instructions (provided by meeting organizers) have information which is vital to planning, such as size, location, length of time for viewing, information to be included, and often layout suggestions.

For planning it is essential to know the **poster size**. Do not take it for granted that all posters are six feet wide by four feet tall (two by one-and-a-half meters). Many are eight feet wide by four feet tall; some are four by four; others may be taller than they are wide. The size of the poster is the first indication of how much to limit the information. The size of the poster also determines the layout.

Poster sessions are **located** in hotel halls, in hotel rooms, or in cavernous convention halls, as in the figure below. The noise level may be high and the lighting level low, neither situation being conducive to thoughtful, leisurely perusal of a poster. This is another reason to limit the information.

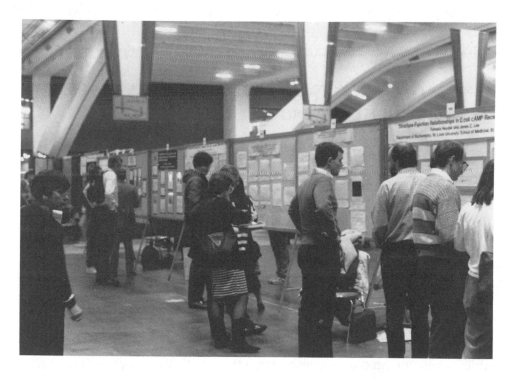

The **length of time for viewing** varies. An hour is the minimum, twenty-three hours the maximum. If the poster will be up for more than an hour, the presenter is not usually expected to be there the whole time. This means that the essential points should be clear and easily understood without personal explanations.

Information in the poster includes the title, the authors' names, and the institution. Sometimes the poster number and the abstract must be added to the title. The title is always positioned at the top of the poster, and instructions usually specify that letter height be one inch (2.5 cm) or larger.

Poster Title

Before sending in the abstract, it is worthwhile to consider how the title will appear on the poster. Lengthy poster titles will discourage the viewer. The first thing that a viewer will see is the title, so it should be brief, informative, and interesting. If a title is enticing or provocative as well, it will attract the viewer's interest.

The following title is lengthy but reasonably informative:

MECHANISM OF AIRWAY CONSTRICTION AND SECRETION EVOKED BY LARYNGEAL ADMINISTRATION OF SO_2 IN DOGS

However, the following version states the conclusion and is shorter and more informative:

EVIDENCE THAT REFLEX EFFECTS OF SO_2 ARE MEDIATED BY AFFERENT ENDINGS IN THE UPPER AIRWAY

But the next version is even shorter and, because it is a question, attracts the viewer's attention:

ARE REFLEX EFFECTS OF SO_2 MEDIATED BY AFFERENT ENDINGS IN THE UPPER AIRWAY?

Even shorter, although perhaps less accurate, is the following:

HOW DOES SO_2 AFFECT THE UPPER AIRWAY?

The first title, when enlarged to one inch high letters, will stretch across five to six feet of width. With the addition of names of authors and institution, the height of the title will be at least six inches. A long title, large enough to be read from twenty feet, will overwhelm the poster.

Abstract

Many meetings specify that abstracts be posted. However, the information in the abstract should also be on the poster in a large, easy to read, organized form. An enlarged abstract will add nothing to the poster.

POSTER WITH ABSTRACT

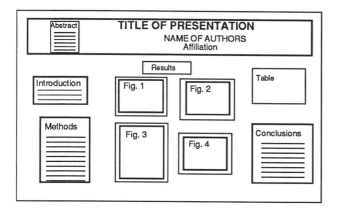

This is a suggested layout that might be included with the poster instructions. The space allotted to the abstract is in the range of nine by four inches. Since it is posted at the top of the poster, near the title, and cannot be adequately enlarged, it will not be legible.

The meeting program will usually contain a copy of the abstract which can be read at leisure. It is a waste of time and money to type and enlarge the abstract. Either leave it out or use a photocopy of it.

Rough Layout

In planning the poster, to visualize size and position, sketch a rough plan. This will give a general idea of how much text and how many figures should be included in the poster. This sketch should show approximate positioning and size of figures and text. The square, vertical, or horizontal shapes of your figures and text begin to evolve in a rough layout.

ROUGH SKETCH

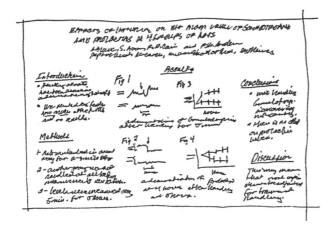

The poster dimensions are approximately 4 by 6 feet, and information is organized into broad topics. The shapes of pre-existing figures are roughly drawn.

In the rough sketch, start to distill your ideas into only the most important points. Decide which one or two points you want the viewer to understand.

Do not try to increase the number of figures or amount of text by making text and figures smaller or by squeezing them together. If the poster is hard to read or cluttered, it will be ineffective. Look again at the information to see what further cuts may be made. Be ruthless and single-minded. <u>Never lose sight of the few points you want to emphasize</u>.

It takes intelligence, even brilliance, to condense and focus information into a clear, simple presentation that will be read and remembered. Ignorance and arrogance are shown in a crowded, complicated, hard-to-read poster.

Poster Text

In writing papers, thoughts are expressed in paragraphs full of sentences which are often long and complex. This verbose kind of writing for a poster causes the viewer to struggle to find the core idea. Plan the poster text in short, simple, separate statements. This allows the viewer to scan the text quickly and easily for the important points.

PARAGRAPH	SEPARATE STATEMENTS
Low concentrations of SO_2 cause bronchoconstriction in asthmatic patients. Since low concentrations of SO_2 may be totally absorbed in the upper airways and since the upper airways appear to be very sensitive to SO_2, we have explored the possibility that SO_2 evokes reflex effects by engaging afferent nerves in the upper airways.	Bronchoconstriction in asthmatic patients is caused by SO_2 in low concentrations. Upper airways are sensitive to and totally absorb low concentrations of SO_2. We explored the possibility that SO_2 engages afferent nerves in the upper airways.

The text on the right can be understood much more quickly than the paragraph on the left because the statements are separated and simplified. Key words such as "Bronchoconstriction" should be put first. Not only does this make it easier to scan text quickly, but it emphasizes important information.

Text for a poster usually includes an introduction or background, methods, results and conclusions. Since the type must be large, you will have to cut down the amount of information. Text should also be titled in order to make the different sections under discussion immediately clear.

TEXT TITLE

INTRODUCTION

SO$_2$ in low concentrations causes bronchoconstriction in asthmatic patients.

Upper airways are sensitive to and totally absorb low concentrations of SO$_2$.

We explored the possibility that SO$_2$ engages afferent nerves in the upper airways.

For quick identification, text should have a title. If each section of text is titled, the flow of information on the poster becomes more apparent.

Here the first statement emphasizes low concentrations of SO$_2$.

Text should be around one quarter inch high (24 point or larger). Following is an example of text size which will give you an idea of how much information may be included in a given space. The title is 36 point bold; the text is 30 point plain.

Try viewing both of these pages from three feet. Even those with perfect eyesight will have to admit that the large lettering on the opposite page can be read much more quickly and easily than the small print.

Remember that many in your audience have reached the "bifocal age" and have difficulties focusing on small type.

INTRODUCTION

Bronchoconstriction in asthmatic patients is caused by SO_2 in low concentrations.

Upper airways are sensitive to and totally absorb low concentrations of SO_2.

We explored the possibility that SO_2 engages afferent nerves in the upper airways.

Text of this size may come as a shock to those who persist in thinking of posters as enlarged papers. Most posters that you will see in meetings have text that is too small and too complex.

This text can be read without strain from three to five feet. Viewers will be drawn by its simplicity and size to scan your text quickly for core ideas.

The font in the sample text is Helvetica, a simple, clean, and legible type face. It is a sans-serif font which means that it lacks the fine lines attached to the extremities of the letters. The title is bold (thick), and the body of the text is plain (thin). This is an excellent font to use for posters since it is easy to read, does not distract from the information, and yet is good looking.

If a serif type such as Times is used, it should be used consistently throughout the poster. This book is printed in a serif type (note the extra lines on the letters). A serif type is said to be easier to read in extensive, small type, but in the large, economical text of a good poster, there is no difference in ease of reading.

Save the use of bold labels for special emphasis, such as the title. Text which is all bold becomes strident and tiring to read. It also overshadows the figures.

DOES THE POSTER DISCOURAGE THE VIEWER?

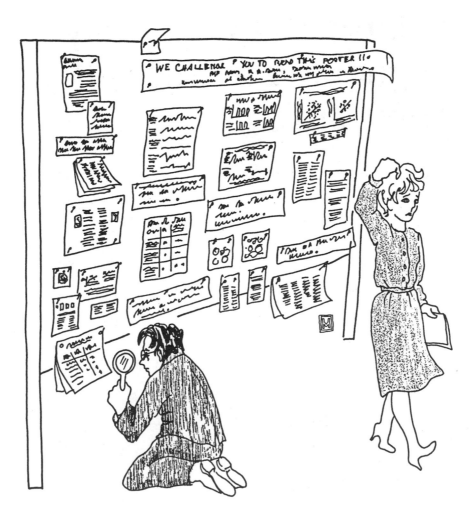

Figures

Figures are more impressive than text on a poster. The poster medium is made for pictures.
Since we learn much more quickly and easily from pictures than from words, use figures to
tell the story and plan the poster around the figures.

Drawings will attract the viewer. They hold the viewer's attention and communicate vividly
and memorably. They are especially effective in describing methods.

METHODS DRAWING

FIGURE 1

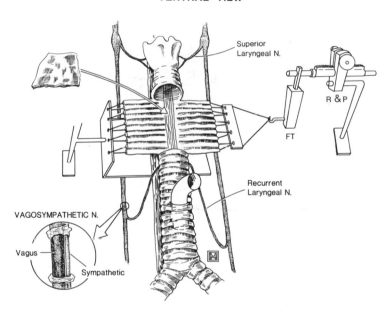

The tracheal segment is connected to a force transducer (FT) and adjusted by
rack and pinion (R & P). The metal plate under the cut trachea prevents
disturbance of the laryngeal nerve branches. The sympathetic nerve is isolated
and surrounded by stimulating electrodes, and contraction is induced by
acetycholine applied to gauze.

This drawing shows an experimental preparation of the trachea. Although it was designed for a paper,
it could be enlarged to make an effective poster figure which could take the place of a long description
of methods. A title and brief explanation of abbreviations and procedure is effectively shown directly
under the drawing.

Graphs must be large. A standard eight and one half by eleven inches is a minimum size. Axis labels should not be less than 24 point. Below is a graph enlarged to a size which is easy to see from three to four feet. Because of the necessarily large size, information on graphs should be limited and labels should be short.

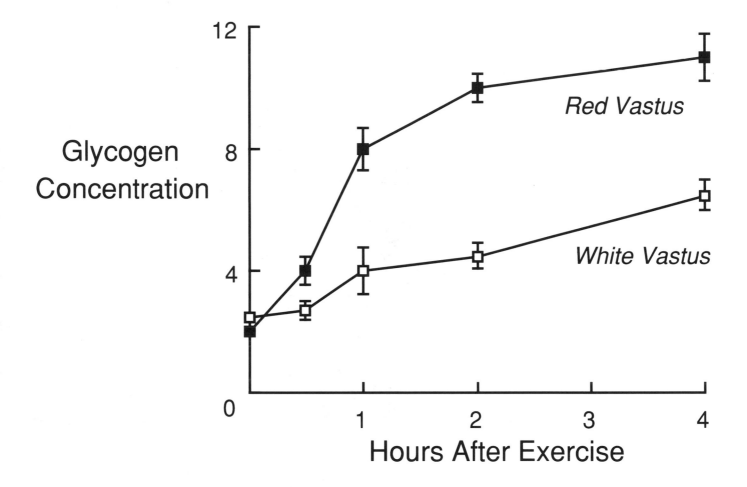

This graph shows the minimum size labels that are easily read from a distance. This figure would be even better if it were turned sideways on the 8.5 by 11 inch page and enlarged still more.

Figures should be numbered prominently for ease of identification and flow of information throughout the poster. If the figure is referred to in the text, it may then be referred to by number. If the figure number reference in the text is made prominent by being bold, all upper case, or larger, it facilitates cross reference of text to figure, figure to text.

A concise figure explanation under the figure may be helpful in clarifying it. In a short statement, details which were left out of the text may be included.

NUMBERED FIGURE WITH LEGEND

FIGURE 1

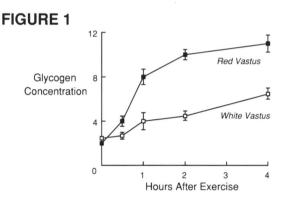

After a swim to exhaustion, glycogen replenishment in skeletal muscle was measured.

The figure number here will make the sequence of information clear. The text underneath clarifies or emphasizes the point and makes it a satisfying, integrated figure.

Poster Layout

A poster should be organized so that the progression of information is clear, keeping in mind that we read from top to bottom and left to right. Important information should be at eye level. The top of the poster will contain the title which is usually read on the approach to the poster. The two feet of space below the title is at eye level for most and is the area where information is most easily read.

READABLE SPACE

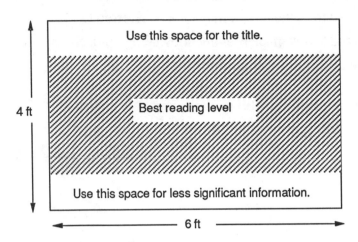

Notice that some of the available poster space falls outside the best reading level. This is another reason for strictly limiting the amount of information. Plan for space around your text and figures. Do not try to cram the whole space with information.

An accurately scaled, penciled layout will help in arranging the information. Make a grid in inches instead of feet, or use graph paper. This serves as a blueprint for relative sizes, juxtapositions, and flow of information.

Plan the poster to be read in sections from left to right and top to bottom. For a six foot wide poster, it is best to divide the space into three or four sections. By doing this, each section can be read while standing in one place. The viewer need only move to the right to read the next section. This is especially practical when there are many people milling around the poster and it makes it possible for several people to read the poster at the same time.

POSTER DIVISIONS

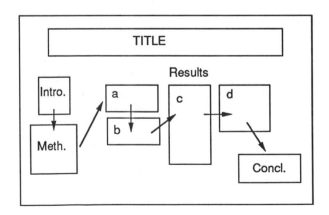

Sections are delineated by grouping of figures and texts and by leaving space between the groups. The arrows indicate one way the eye naturally moves through the poster.

Lay out the poster before the meeting to get some idea of how it will look. Check for consistency of style, terminology, and symbolism. Show it to your colleagues and to scientists outside of your expertise. Ask them and yourself if the poster presents a clear, simple, cohesive message.

Poster Production

There are many ways to prepare and assemble the poster materials, from time-saving, simple, and inexpensive to time-consuming, sophisticated, and expensive. While your own resources may be a limiting factor, the one thing you should not stint on is your time. Even if the poster is produced by a commercial design studio, the time you spend carefully planning and organizing the information will determine its success. The time you spend consulting with the artist and photographer will make a difference. If you produce your own poster, plan to spend several days on it.

Enlargement

The size of **photographic** enlargements is limited only by available photographic paper size. Photographic enlargement is the most faithful to the original. For posters, such enlargements should be printed on a matte surface paper in order to avoid glare and reflection.

A **P.M.T.** is a photomechanical transfer, a positive print made without a negative. It is printed on a matte finish paper and is useful for enlargements up to 18 by 24 inches. Since it requires no negative, it is less expensive than a photographic enlargement. The largest size costs around $20.

Enlargements by **copying machines** are limited to 14 by 17 inches. One-ply bond paper is usually used although other, finer, one-ply papers, such as plate finish bristol, may sometimes be substituted. At 25 ¢ per copy, this is the least expensive kind of enlargement.

Enlargements may be made by **computer** and printed on a laser printer. Although maximum paper size is 8.5 by 14 inches, paper may be spliced together for any size. Print quality is good and for anyone with access to a computer/laser printer, this is a quick, flexible, and inexpensive way to produce title, text, and figures.

Photo murals are enlargements of the whole poster. Individual parts of the poster are pieced together in half or third size and then enlarged to the final size on one large sheet of matte finish photographic paper. This is rolled up for transport to the meeting, then unrolled and tacked to the poster surface.

The maximum width of the paper (which comes in rolls), is 42 inches, slightly less than a four foot poster height. A photo mural requires a negative which costs around nine dollars, and the print, itself, costs around four dollars a square foot, so that a 3.5 by 5.5 foot blow-up will cost around $90.

Text Production

Type-written text is not a viable alternative for posters unless it is enlarged. However, to go from typewriter size text to a reasonable poster size means an enlargement of 400 to 500 %, often with extreme loss of quality.

Text which is **type-set** results in enlargements of excellent quality, but entails not only the typesetter's charge, but an additional cost of enlargement.

Computer-typed text, printed and enlarged by the laser printer, is the best alternative. The print quality is good and changes in text and enlargement may be easily made. A word-processing program is most flexible for this purpose, although some drawing programs provide good text options.

Trimming and Mounting

Trimming of figures, text, and title may be necessary to save space or to splice pages together. This can be done with an accurate paper cutter or sharp knife against a metal ruler.

For the most basic production, the enlarged, separate text figures and title can be taken to the meeting and tacked onto the assigned board according to plan. However, mounting the separate parts on light board adds body, durability, and color.

Material for mounting may be one of the following:

1. Poster board and railroad board are lightweight boards that come in a variety of colors.

2. Mat board is heavier and also available in many colors. It is harder to cut than the lighter boards.

3. Cover stock and construction paper are heavy papers, easy to cut and available in an array of colors. Although these papers are not as durable as heavier boards, they are easier to transport since they are thinner and weigh less.

To mount the poster to the backing board, use a **spray adhesive** such as 3M Photo Mount™. This coats the paper evenly and is quick and easy to use. The item to be glued is placed face down on newspaper or other throw-away material. This prevents excess spray glue from covering the floor or table surface. The back of the item is sprayed, then pressed into position on the backing material.

Rubber cement takes more time to apply and is not as smooth as spray adhesive. Glue Stic™ is handy for small items, but also takes time to apply.

Poster Backgrounds

The poster surface provided at most meetings is tan cork board or white composition board. They are neutral to ugly looking. The white background swallows and absorbs the white paper on which your poster parts are printed. In this case, a color background is essential for contrast, emphasis and clarity.

Often a professionally done poster utilizes a **mat board background** that covers the entire poster space. Figures are mounted on accurately pieced together boards so that when they are tacked to the meeting board, the pieces form a solid colored background. This is time consuming and requires expertise in accurate positioning of figures and cutting of boards. The result, however is a consistent background color that frames the poster text and figures and unites them into a cohesive whole.

Another possibility for background color is **Velcro™ material** cut to the poster size and tacked to the meeting board along the edges. When pieces of adhesive loop tape are applied to the backs of the poster parts, they can be quickly mounted on the Velcro-covered board and just as quickly changed around and taken down.

There are also heavy **seamless papers** in 53 and 107 inch widths in many colors. These papers may be cut to poster board size and tacked to the board. This provides a smooth color background for tacking poster items.

Color

Color is a great asset in posters. Color backgrounds frame and unify the poster parts. Color keys used consistently throughout the poster make information easier to follow. In addition, color is pleasing and attractive to the viewer.

If possible, use color backing; apply color to columns in bar graphs with color markers or color film; use color paper for arrows; use color transfer letters for short labels; use color photographs and drawings. Just make sure they are large.

Although large photographic color prints are expensive, less expensive color prints can be made using the color photostat process or the color copier.

The maximum size for a **color photostat** is 11 by 16.5 inches and maximum enlargement is 200%. A color slide may be enlarged to this maximum size. In this process, the range of colors is fairly subtle and the background will be a neutral color similar to that of a photographic print. A maximum sized stat costs around $23.

The **color copier** uses a laser printing process and enlarges a maximum of 400%. Maximum paper size for printing is 11 by 17 inches. Each copy costs around $4. Color quality in these prints is brighter and more artificial, tending to exaggerate yellow, but the background is the pure white of the bond paper used in this process.

Transport

Most meetings are held away from home and entail plane travel with its attendant baggage and space complications. Consider this when deciding how to produce the poster. For easy transport, the poster should be lightweight and compact enough to take on the plane. Checking the poster with baggage risks losing or damaging it.

A photo mural can be carried rolled into a four foot mailing tube.

Posters mounted on large sections of mat board are awkward to carry, but sections may be cut and taped so that they can be folded to a more compact size. If they will not fit into a briefcase or large envelope, at least cover them with heavy wrapping paper to avoid dirt and damage.

Better yet, use a heavy, corrugated mailing box. These come in a 23 by 13 by $2^1/_2$ inch size and can be located under "Boxes - Corrugated & Fiber" in the yellow pages.

Separate poster items should be planned to fit into a briefcase or heavy box. Velcro™ material can be folded and put into a suitcase or box, and seamless paper backing can be rolled into a mailing tube.

Poster Purpose

Communication of one or two ideas should be the purpose of the poster. The purpose of a poster is **not** vanity or ambition. Unfortunately, in the crowded, noisy, poorly-lit halls for poster sessions, there is often very little communication at all.

Scientists could learn from advertisers. Compare the average scientific poster with an advertisement in a scientific journal. No matter what you think of the value of advertisements, they communicate effectively. Advertisers spend large sums of money, thought, and time to present limited information concisely, clearly, and attractively.

Observe and think about what communicates to you, what communicates to your colleagues. If you genuinely desire to teach others through your poster, you will not be afraid to be simple, clear and creative.

12

USING AN ILLUSTRATOR

Art and science, far from being exclusive, have a long history of symbiotic, fluid, and rich relationships. Vesalius, daVinci, Audubon, and Beatrix Potter are famous personifications of this marriage of science and art.

A medical or scientific illustrator is an expert at making drawings, diagrams, tables, and graphs. Ideally, an illustrator's expertise should be available to all scientists. An artist's way of seeing scientific information and rendering that information into effective visual presentation can be of great benefit to scientists.

Having done the research, the scientist expects details, accuracy, and flexibility of data presentation. The artist, concerned with communicating understanding of a clear message, looks for visual accuracy in communicating the large story the data tell and the visual details which will display that message best. Collaboration between artist and scientist, if only by consultation, is often the preferred way to do figures.

A trained scientific illustrator is more proficient than a scientist in some areas of illustration, and some figures are more efficiently done by an illustrator.

For complex drawings or diagrams, an illustrator is a necessity. For tables, charts and graphs, an illustrator can save time. An illustrator can help plan and can evaluate and make suggestions for figures done by hand or by computer.

An illustrator's skill in drawing and design can turn an adequate figure into a clearer and more interesting figure

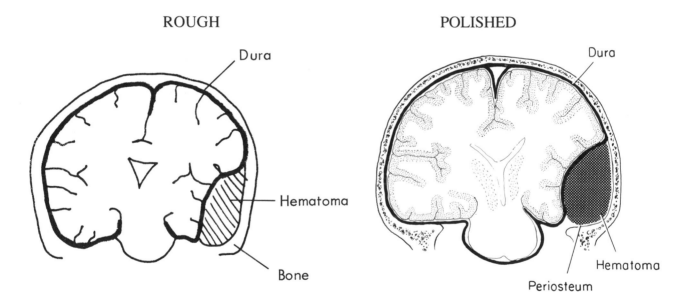

Both of these drawings show blood collected between the dura and periosteum, forming a hematoma. On the left, the general area of the hematoma and rough configuration of the dura are apparent. But the artist's rendering on the right is more exact and contains more detail. It is also visually more interesting.

An illustrator can help communicate by visually synthesizing, clarifying, and simplifying your ideas. An illustrator can help plan the figures by presenting choices and suggesting alternatives. An illustrator can serve as a consultant for figures made on the computer.

Communicate With the Illustrator

Before seeing an illustrator, take time to plan and organize your ideas. Start this planning well before the deadline.

- Know what you want to show in the drawing. Decide on priorities.
- Check journal, poster, or meeting instructions for size and final form.
- Check for accuracy of ideas or data. Discuss rough ideas with colleagues or co-authors.

Provide the illustrator with the following information:

- The meaning and significance of the figure.
    The illustrator must understand at least the general nature of the information in order to suggest ways of presentation.
    Take advantage of an illustrator's expertise by asking for such suggestions.
- What it will be used for.
- The deadline.
- Raw data or rough drafts of information or ideas.
- Any reference material which will be needed.

Be aware of the steps involved in drawing:

- Research and/or on-site sketching.
- Decision about the technique to be used. For example:
    Pen and ink reproduces well in journals and is economical to print.
    Carbon dust, pencil, watercolor, or airbrush tone rendering is smooth and most realistic. These techniques may take more time than pen and ink and in reproduction has a grey background. It is effective for slides but is more expensive for journal reproduction since a half-tone must be made.
    Color paper, color film, color pencil, pastel, watercolor, or airbrush rendering are effective for slides and posters but are expensive for publication.

- Several sketches before the final sketch.
- The final drawing.
- Possible changes anytime in the process.

Budget more time and money for drawings and color work than for black and white graphs. Check all work carefully and allow time for changes, additions, and corrections. Allow five working days for photography of the final art work.

The Illustrator and the Computer

The widespread use of the computer for charts and graphs has been a boon for the illustrator as well as the researcher. The time and tedium involved in hand-done, repetitious graphs have been eliminated. Many illustrators can enter the data and plot and print the graph effectively and quickly by computer. An illustrator also brings expertise in design to this exercise which may make the difference between a good or bad graph.

Almost all computer-drawn graphs require visual editing. Visual editing involves observation of what works visually to communicate information. It involves making the educated choices described in *Chapter 7, Kinds of Graphs,* and *Chapter 8, Designing Graphs.* An illustrator can look at the graph below and suggest simple ways to improve it.

ROUGH COMPUTER GRAPH

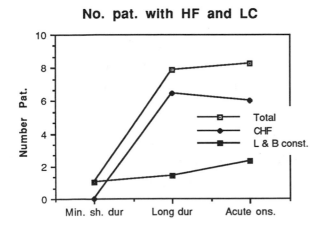

The graph on the left shows the total number of patients who died in a study, broken down into symptoms and kinds of illness. This is an example of information which looks much more complicated than it is. Abbreviated labels are unclear; the y-axis is cluttered with numbers and ticks; the frame around the graph serves no purpose. Above all, a line graph is not the best way to show totals with divisions.

POLISHED COMPUTER GRAPH

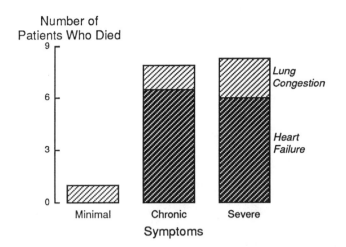

An illustrator could make the changes shown in this graph or could suggest that you make such changes. Here information is shown in a stacked bar graph which shows totals with divisions into the kinds of disease. Labels are written out in simple terms; the y-axis is simplified and the plot frame removed.

The Illustrator as a Resource

An illustrator can describe and demonstrate materials and their uses and can recommend sources for materials and services. Long experience with the assets and limitations of tools and different media make the illustrator a valuable and practical resource.

An artist can be an antidote to the scientist who is so immersed in the work that what seems simple after years of involvement, "must be clear to others". An artist may often be more useful than colleagues in looking at visual material objectively and in assessing whether this material will be understood outside of the scientist's specialized field.

Above all, an artist has an ability to simplify and get to the point visually. This trait is essential for communicating visual material. It is a trait which is often lacking in scientists who are trained in verbal but not visual skills. The artist is trained to observe details and relationships in the context of a cohesive whole picture while the scientist often gets bogged down by details.

13

USING A COMPUTER

Many scientists are finding that, besides being a useful tool for research, computers enable them to do graphs, tables, word slides, and simple diagrams quickly and easily. Personal computers are relatively inexpensive and are easy to learn to use. There are excellent programs for making illustrations on the computer. The computer-done examples in this chapter were all done on the Macintosh Plus computer, printed out on a laser printer, but could also have been done on an MS-DOS machine.

Computer-made diagrams and graphs are certainly within the capabilities of any scientist and use of computers by scientists often helps to clarify ideas and to increase visual perception. The use of computers by scientists for graphics can be a rewarding and enjoyable experience.

Some assets of computer use for preparing illustrations:
- Speed.
- Ease of use.
- Ease of change.
- Possibilities for experimentation.

As with any tool, the end product depends upon the skill of the user. The multiplicity of choices offered in most programs requires that the user have clear goals and know what works to communicate well visually.

Some difficulties of computer use for doing illustrations are:

- Program limitations.

  Old ways of doing a figure may have to be adapted to what the program can provide.

  Nonstandard figures may not fit into one program and may require transfer to another program.

- Computer speed and ease abet a tendency for rush jobs, often resulting in carelessly planned and executed figures.

- Complicated figures and drawings can take a great deal of time.

- A preoccupation with the medium itself may distract from the main goal: to communicate clearly and simply.

A computer is a tool that takes time, practice, and experimentation to get good results. More than that, it takes awareness of the requirements of good illustrations discussed throughout this book. Do not be dazzled by its speed and versatility. Do not let the medium be the message.

Letters, Fonts, and Styles

The fact that the computer program has options for many fonts, sizes, and styles does not mean that all are appropriate to use.

DISTRACTING LABELS	SIMPLE LABELS

ISOLATE OLIGOSACCHARIDES

DIRECT DETECTION OF LOW PICO-
MOLE LEVELS OF CARBOHYDRATES.

SELECTIVE RESOLUTION OF
POSITIONAL ISOMERS.

ANALYSE CARBOHYDRATES

| High resolution ion exchange resins. |
| Pulsed amperometric detector. |

ISOLATE OLIGOSACCHARIDES
  • Direct detection of low-picomole
    levels of carbohydrates.
  • Selective resolution of positional
    isomers.

ANALYSE CARBOHYDRATES
  • High resolution anion exchange resins.
  • Pulsed amperometric detector.

On the left, all labeling is bold. Upper case and mixed upper and lower case labels are used without purpose. The various styles (outline, shadow, underline, italic) say to the viewer, "Look how much the computer can do." Scientific information is not communicated here. On the right, font is plain and sans-serif ; upper case is used for the two main headings. Information under the headings is upper and lower case and clarified by bullets and by being inset. Here the computer was used to clarify and simplify information.

Because it is easy to generate good-looking text, do not get carried away. Hand-written text which is brief, well organized, and carefully planned may be preferable to a poorly planned, disorganized figure no matter how sophisticated its execution.

Use Computer Options to Simplify and Organize

For flow charts, tables, and diagrams, the computer offers almost limitless possibilities for rearrangement and variation of the composition. Take advantage of these assets to make the figure more easily understood. Use these assets to organize and simplify.

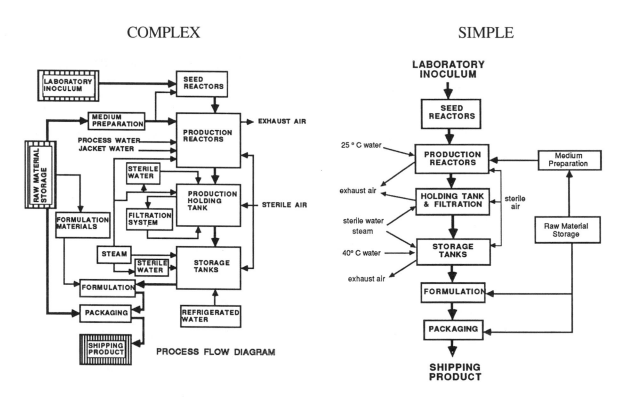

The flow chart on the left is cluttered and complicated. All the labels are the same size and style and there is no focus for attention. To go from inoculum to product in this chart is to go through a baffling maze. On the right , the pathway from inoculum to product is straight and easy to follow. By the use of large, bold labels, the emphasis is on this pathway. The plain, upper and lower case labels to the right of the pathway are less emphatic and the smaller, unboxed labels to the left are least emphatic. Rearrangement of the flow into three columns of unequal importance has clarified the information and eliminated some repetition and clutter.

The computer is a flexible tool ready to do your bidding. But it will not plan, simplify, and emphasize information unless you tell it to.

Computer Drawings and Diagrams

There are many computer programs which can be used to make simple and complex drawings and diagrams. Among them are Mac Paint, Mac Draw, Cricket Draw, Adobe Illustrator, and Aldus Freehand for the Macintosh. Good programs for MS-DOS computers are Corel Draw, Arts and Letters, Micrografx Designer, and Adobe Illustrator. Some programs, such as Mac Paint and Mac Draw, are easy to learn while others such as Adobe Illustrator and Corel Draw are more sophisticated and difficult to learn.

However, use of a computer for a complex drawing may be time-consuming no matter which program is used. A hand-drawn figure may be quicker and just as effective.

HAND DRAWN   COMPUTER DRAWN

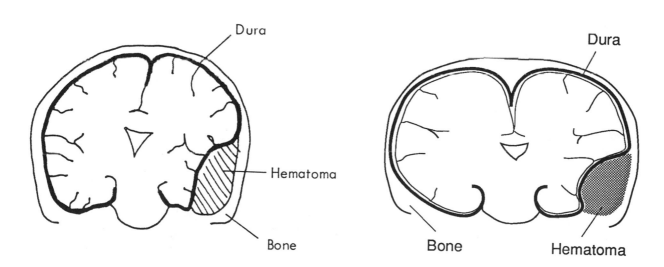

The drawing on the left was sketched in pencil, then overdrawn with a thick and a thin point felt-tipped pen. It was drawn to the size shown and the labels were typed. It took about an hour. The computer drawing was done using the Adobe Illustrator program and took an hour and a half. Much more detail is possible in this program, but would add to the time involved.

Although drawings take time, it may be time well spent if it helps you to clarify and focus your own ideas. Most of us are born artists, largely untrained. Doing drawings by pencil or computer may enable you to look at the information with fresh eyes. It can lead to a different way of thinking about the information and even suggest further paths to take.

Laser print from the computer has even, crisp lines and many copies of equal quality may be made. Changes and additions can be quickly and easily made. The size and relative dimensions of the computer drawing may be varied and it can be used in combination with other computer drawings.

If you do not need these advantages, and do not expect to use the drawing again, a hand drawn figure may be adequate and may save a little time. Also, some kinds of drawings are more suitable than others for the computer. Any drawing which requires strict accuracy or much repetition is much better done on the computer.

MOTIF AND REPETITION

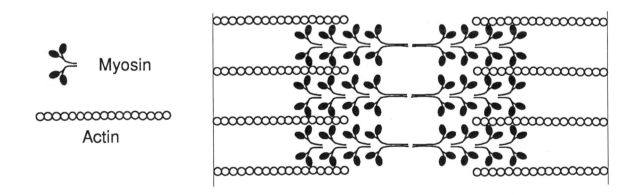

On the left are two motifs, actin and myosin. These may be quickly and accurately repeated to form the diagram on the right. Time and care spent on a motif to be repeated is well spent. The above figure was done on the Adobe Illustrator program.

A diagram which can be changed and extended is often valuable for communicating. This is easily done with a computer.

DIAGRAM   WITH CHANGE AND SUBTRACTION

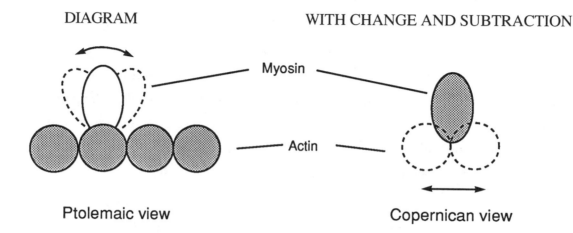

Ptolemaic view   Copernican view

In the view on the left, the myosin moves while the actin is stationary, analogous to the sun moving around the earth. On the right the myosin is stationary while the actin moves (earth moves around the sun). The basis of these diagrams is the ellipse and the circle. Lines, stippling and positions have been changed and circles and ellipses added and subtracted. Both diagrams were done in the Cricket Draw program.

Most drawing programs offer options for exact rotating, reflecting, duplicating, and shading. These and other options such as variations of line thickness and style present numerous artistic and organizational choices. To make the right choices:

- Know exactly what you want to show.
- Try various ways of showing it. (The computer provides quick and easy ways to change.)
- Observe the differences carefully.
- If you are not sure which way works best, ask colleagues, artists, and friends for their opinion.

Bit Mapped vs Vector-Based Graphics

There are two kinds of computer-generated graphics, bit-mapped and vector-based. A discussion of the differences between the two may help decide which program to use.

A **bit-mapped** image is formed on the computer screen by a series of digital bits or square pixels. When printed, each of these bits corresponds to a printed pixel on the paper. Mac Paint or Paint Brush are bit-mapped programs. Diagonal and curved lines in bit-mapped programs show noticeable stair-steps and appear jagged and somewhat crude. Enlargement of this kind of graphic exaggerates the "jaggies".

While some designers use this jagged look to advantage, before deciding to use a bit-mapped program, decide whether it is appropriate for the subject.

Vector-based graphics (sometimes called line art or objects graphics) are mathematical descriptions of an object. These mathematical descriptions are represented on the screen by a series of dots. Output to the printed page is also a result of interpretation of the mathematical description to dots on the page. Diagonal and curved lines are correspondingly smoother and enlargements do not suffer deterioration. Mac Draw and Adobe Illustrator are vector-based programs.

Drawing programs permit freehand drawing; graphing programs operate from data sheets to convert numbers to graphs. There is limited freehand drawing and annotation permitted in graphing programs.

Computer Generated Graphs

The most widespread and helpful use for the computer is making graphs. A good graphing program offers flexible and speedy data input, a variety of kinds of graphs, and options for label, axes, and symbol changes. Programs used for graph making are Cricket Graph for the Macintosh, and Harvard Graphics and Slide Write Plus for MS-DOS. Also, most spreadsheets, such as Lotus 1-2-3, Quattro, and Excel, have limited graphing programs.

Input of data on the computer requires typing, proofing, and possible changes and rearranging of data. Graphing requires the selection of axes and standard errors. In addition, changes are usually required in the axes lengths and units, label content, size, and style. You may also want to change the shape of the graph, save the format, or print it in a different size or alignment. Since you will probably discover errors or want to add information, you could easily generate a half dozen printed versions.

All of this takes time. Plan to spend an hour or more to make a publication-quality graph. In compensation, however, changes and additions may be made quickly.

Below are some steps in making a graph using the Cricket Graph program on the Macintosh computer.

DATA INPUT

	Minutes	Pre-resection	3 - 4 weeks	6 - 7 weeks
1	0.000	4.600	4.500	4.800
2	1.000	3.500	3.750	1.750
3	2.000	3.750	4.400	3.650
4	3.000	3.800	4.600	4.500
5	4.000	3.900	4.800	5.200
6	5.000	3.950	4.800	5.100
7	6.000	4.000	4.700	5.200
8	7.000	4.100	4.600	5.100
9	8.000	4.200	4.500	4.900
10	9.000	4.170	4.300	5.000

Data may be entered by row (across the page) or by column (down the page). Corrections and additions are easily made. Often data which are originally entered from the experiment directly onto the computer may be transferred to a graphing program. With large quantities of information this saves a great deal of time.

UNEDITED GRAPH

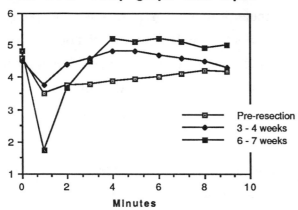

This is the graph showing the program default format. Notice that the axes are longer than necessary and have too many ticks. Labels are not accurate or complete and symbols are not clearly distinct. There is an unnecessary plot frame and the shape of the graph may be unsuitable.

EDITED GRAPH

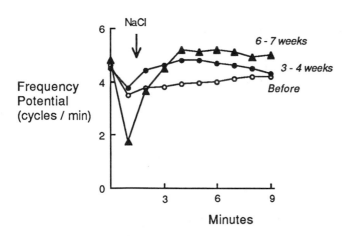

In this graph, the plot frame and the legend are removed. Labels are changed and added. Label font is plain and compatible with the laser printer; size and style are varied to emphasize priorities. Symbols are simplified to solid and open, and the width of the graph is compressed to accommodate horizontal y-axis labels.

Making changes which fit the information is the most time-consuming but most important part of making a graph that is clear and conveys the message.

Computer Print Out

Both drawing and graphing programs permit output to **laser printers**. It is the laser printer which makes computer drawings and graphs viable for publication, slides, and posters. The quality of line and tone is good at around 300 dots per inch.

Post Script is the language used to drive most laser printers, so that work done on the computer is converted by Post Script descriptions to fit the printed page. Although Post Script was developed originally as a typesetting language, it also permits output of vector-based graphics from both the Macintosh and MS-DOS computers to the compatible laser printer. In addition, Post Script files also transfer to the typesetter's Linotronic printer. This printer generates 1200 to 2400 dots per inch and produces very fine quality print.

Use of good quality **paper** or film will affect the quality of the printed copy. The Linotronic printer uses a smooth, light-sensitive film but it is possible to substitute special papers for the usual bond paper in the computer laser printer. Pro-Tech is a computer paper made by the James River Corporation in various qualities: 25% cotton bond, parchment, and coated, heavier paper for crisp, clean print. For information, the toll-free number is: 1-800-521-5035.

The multitude of choices facing you in making graphs are both artistic and organizational. So, knowing what you want to say, trying various ways to say it and observing which works best for what you want to say, are as important for making graphs on the computer as for drawings.

14

DRAWING BY HAND

Since illustrators and computers are not available to all researchers, the ability to draw figures by hand is a valuable skill. Processes such as mounting and labeling gels and physiological tracings are not difficult to do. The process of making graphs becomes easy with practice, indeed, a relaxing change.

If you decide to do figures by hand, set aside time to do them well. If you have never done diagrams or graphs by hand you need as much information as possible. Consult books, chartists, artists, and people you know who have experience in doing their own figures by hand. You need patience and practice in addition to information.

Below are descriptions of useful and simple processes that anyone can do with a minimum of equipment and time. Tools and materials are also described. You may find that if you do not make your own figures frequently, tools and materials may be mislaid and your familiarity with them may have to be refreshed by practice before you begin. Take this into consideration when setting aside time to do your figures. Expect that you will make mistakes, so plan time for changes and additions.

Trim, Mount, and Label Tracings

Physiologic tracings are usually recorded on graph paper. Most of the time you will want to use only selected parts of the tracing to illustrate your point. You may want to eliminate single lines or whole sections of multiple tracings. You may want to combine scattered parts of the tracing. Also, for clarity of communication, tracings should have scales and brief labels. Even if a computer directly prints out physiologic recordings, it may be easier to combine, eliminate, and label parts by hand.

Tools and materials* which you will need for this are:

- A T-square, preferably metal.

- A drawing board against which a T-square will fit and on which tracings may be cut.

- A triangle, preferably metal.

- A cutting knife (e.g. #1 X-acto knife) with #11 blades.

- Two-ply, plate finish bristol paper.

- Masking tape.

- A technical pen, (e.g. Rotring or Koh-I-Noor Rapidograph) in a fine point size. Number 0 (.35 mm) or number 1 (.50 mm) are good sizes.

- Black drawing ink, (e.g. Pelikan) and liquid pen cleaner (e.g. Rapido-eze or Speedball).

- Sheets of transfer lettering (e.g. Letraset or Chart Pak).

- Spray adhesive (e.g. 3M Photo Mount).

---

* Materials listed are available in art and drafting supply stores, and in some stationery stores. Also various catalogs are available for mail orders. For Flax Artist Materials Catalog, call: 800-546-7778.

Before beginning, use a photocopy machine to make practice copies. A photocopy machine is also valuable for making the fine lines of the tracing darker and thicker so that you may want to mount the copy rather than the original. A photocopy machine will also drop out light colored grid lines and some machines will reduce or enlarge the tracings.

PHOTOCOPY FOR PRACTICE

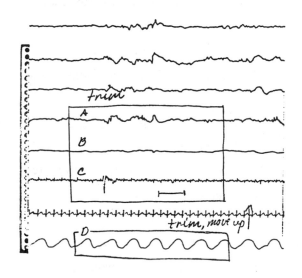

If elements of the tracing are to be eliminated or combined, do this first on a copy to see if this is what you want. You can also label the copy in pencil to get an idea of position, size and content. Make mistakes and alterations on a copy rather than on the original tracing.

Trim the tracing

- Align the tracing with the T-square and tape it to the board.
- Using the cutting knife and a sharp blade, make horizontal cuts along the T-square.
- Place the triangle against the T-square for a perfect right angle. Make vertical cuts along the triangle.
- Mark the backs of the cut tracings for ease in mounting.

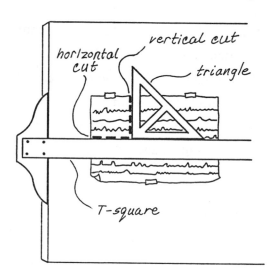

To avoid making scratches on the board with the cutting knife, use a cutting mat. These are available in many sizes and allow the knife to bite into the rubber-hard surface of the mat without showing cut marks.

Mount the Tracing

- Tape the bristol paper to the board.
- Loosely position the cut tracings as desired on the board and mark their final positions lightly with pencil.
- Using the T-square and triangle, pencil in light vertical and horizontal lines indicating the desired positions of the trimmed tracings.
- Lay the tracings face down on newspapers which have been spread out to protect floor or desk surfaces from excess spray adhesive. Spray the backs of the tracings following directions on the can.
- Position the sprayed tracings along the lines marked on the bristol paper. If a tracing is misaligned, lift it carefully from the paper and reposition.
- After tracings are in position, cover them with clean paper and rub them down with a thumb nail or a burnisher. (3M makes a 4 inch wide burnisher which is excellent for this purpose.)
- Erase all pencil lines. If there is adhesive on or around the tracings, it may be removed with a gum eraser or small amounts of rubber cement thinner.

Mark Units

Since the lines of tracings are fine, their unit markings and labels should also be fine so that they will not compete with or overwhelm the tracings themselves. Use a fine tipped technical pen (#0 or #1 point) for scale markings, axes lines, and tick marks. This kind of pen must be held perpendicularly to the paper between thumb and forefinger. The pen should be angled away from the T-square or triangle to prevent ink from running under them. Or put layers of masking tape on the bottom sides of the T-square and triangle to lift them from the paper. Take the time to practice drawing straight lines against the T-square and triangle.

PEN AND INK

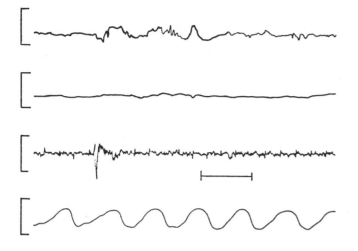

On the left is the trimmed, mounted tracing. Vertical unit scales and a horizontal time scale were first marked with pencil, then traced with a #0 pen and Pelikan brand drawing ink. Cut lines, faint grids and differences in papers do not reproduce in photocopies or high-contrast film.

Pens have to be kept clean and must be handled carefully. If you prefer not to use pen and ink, other options are:

- Pressure sensitive graphic **tape** in a #1 point size (.35 mm). This may be positioned on your marked pencil line and cut to the appropriate length.

- **Transfer lines** (e.g. Letraset) are available in various thicknesses (#83-106), or .5 point only (#4269), or 1 point (#4271). These lines may be cut through the plastic sheet in any length and rubbed onto the penciled lines with the point of a pencil or a special burnisher (sometimes referred to as a spatula) for this purpose. Use nonphoto blue Berol Prismacolor or Berol Verithin pencil lines for marking postiton lines since they do not need to be erased. Nonphoto blue is a particular shade of blue which does not reproduce on film. Erasure of lines near transfer labels risks removing the labels.

Label the Tracing

Transfer type comes in various sizes, fonts, and styles. Helvetica Light or Helvetica Medium is a sans serif font which is readable and good looking. A light or fine-lined font works best for fine-lined tracings. For an average 81/2 by 11 inch tracing, 18 point size works well. However, it is wise to buy several sizes: 18-point for the main labels, 14-point for numbers, 24-point for titles. Stick to one font for consistency and make sure you will have enough of the required letters and numbers.

Before applying the labels, use the T-square to draw a light blue pencil line slightly below the label position. There is a dashed line below the letters on the sheet. Align this dashed line along the pencil line while you position the first letter. With your finger, press the letter into contact with the paper. Then rub back and forth across the letter with the pencil point or spatula using light pressure. Peel back the sheet and the letter is transferred. Do the same for the subsequent letters until the word is complete. When the word or sentence is finished, cover it with the blue backing paper and burnish or rub it with the spatula or your thumb nail.

TRANSFER LABELS

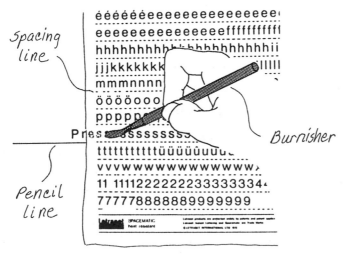

The sheet of transfer lettering shown on the left is Letraset brand, Helvetica Light font. The X-acto spoon burnisher shown is especially helpful in transferring large labels. An old ball-point pen or a pencil works well for letters under 30 point size.

To remove a label, cover it with masking tape and rub it down. The label will stick to the tape when you remove it.

The dashed lines below the letters are actually marks for spacing. If you need help spacing the letters in a word, transfer the right hand space bar (dash) under the letter along with the first letter. Butt the left hand space bar of the next letter against the previous space bar. Transfer this letter and its right-hand space bar and do the same for the following letters of the word.

If rubbing does not transfer the letters, or if the transferred letters appear cracked or uneven, it may be because the sheet is old. You can try lightly rubbing the letter on the blue backing sheet before transferring it, and holding the Letraset sheet in position while carefully peeling it back. Or, to spare yourself frustration, throw away the old sheet and buy a new one.

You may find that you use up certain letters or numbers quickly, leaving the rest of the sheet unused. This makes Letraset an expensive form of labeling (the cost is now around $12 per sheet). It is also time-consuming, especially if labels must be centered. To center accurately, roughly trace the letters of the word or sentence in pencil on a tissue overlay. Position the traced word or sentence on your paper and mark the beginning position for transfer.

Other possibilities for labeling are the lettering systems such as **Leroy** or the **Kroy** labeling machine. The Leroy system uses a scriber and various size templates to ink directly on the paper. The Kroy machine prints labels on adhesive backed tape which is then cut and positioned on the paper.

LEROY SYSTEM

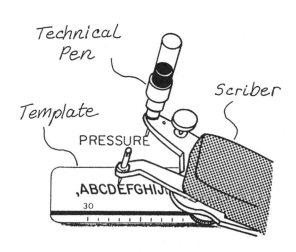

With practice, this system becomes a versatile, quick, and inexpensive way to label. Although the font is unchangeable, the style may be changed to italics, and pens may be interchanged to produce thicker or thinner lines.

KROY LETTERING MACHINE

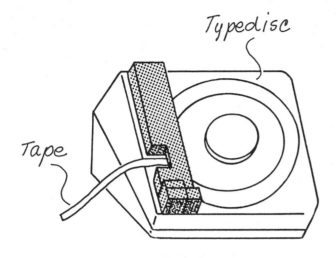

Typedisc

Tape

The Kroy machine might be compared to a typewriter. Characters are automatically spaced and aligned. A carbon impression of each character is pressure fused to an adhesive-backed tape. The tape backing paper must be removed before it is applied to the desired position. It can be repositioned and removed easily. Several kinds of tape are available, including color tape. Each typedisc represents one style in one size.

While centering is easy in the Kroy system, the edges of the tape will show in continuous tone photographic reproduction. Centering is a problem with the Leroy system, but it reproduces well for any film. Both systems have a high initial cost which can be justified if you do frequent labeling.

Computer-generated labels printed on a laser printer look professional and may be printed in all the usual sizes and fonts. The back of the labeled sheets can be spray-glued and cut out , positioned, and rubbed onto the figure. Or use a glue stick on the cut-out label and affix.

For frequent gluing of small items like labels, a hand-held waxer is useful. It heats wax electrically and rolls out a thin coat onto paper. Once the waxed item is pressed into position, it stays well but is also easy to peel off and reapply if changes are required.

Trim, Mount, and Label Gels

The process described above for tracings may be used also for photographs of gels. It is a good idea to photocopy the gels and trim and label the photocopy to experiment with spacing and labels.

Since photographs of gels are generally no larger than 5 by 7 inches, labels should be small. Use Letraset point sizes 10, 12 and 14. If you use more numbers than letters, you might experiment with sheets of numbers only. Numbers in Helvetica font come in various point size but in medium thickness only. If you can find sheets of numbers in Futura Medium, this is a lighter type face than the other fonts, yet goes well with them.

Indicator lines may be drawn with a fine point technical pen or rubbed on from sheets of transfer lines. Remember to leave space around the trimmed gel photos so that two negatives may be made of the final gel. See *Chapter 4, Photographs.*

Draw and Label Graphs

Sometimes it is quicker to draw a graph by hand than by computer, especially if you have already plotted it on graph paper. Detached axes, composite graphs, special curve fits, and graphs with special axes all usually require transfer to another drawing program for additional time-consuming changes.

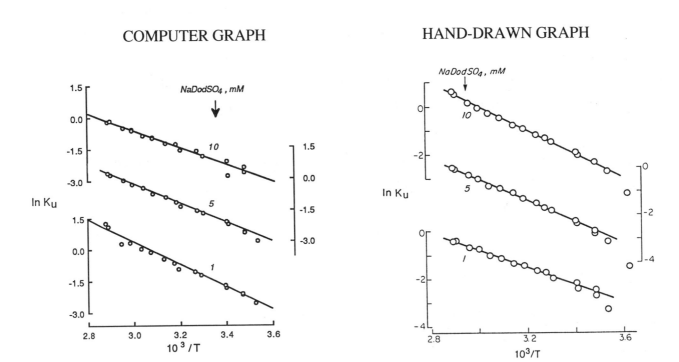

The computer drawn graph on the left is three graphs with data entered for each, and each one plotted separately. Although some time was saved by using the same format for each graph, all three had to be transferred to a drawing program. Total time to do this is close to two hours. The similar hand-drawn graph on the right can be done in less time if you have had some practice drawing graphs.

Sometimes it is satisfying to spend time working directly on paper, using hand tools. Often the result of a hand-drawn graph will be more pleasing. Axes lines and ticks on hand-drawn graphs can be variable thicknesses and do not have to be so heavy relative to the other lines. You have more control over symbol size, line styles, and letter spacing. Drawing graphs can be a relaxing change for you which may even be therapeutic.

With practice and proper materials and tools, graphs may be made quickly by hand. Many of the **tools and materials** listed above for mounting and labeling tracings may be used also to make graphs. In addition to the board, T-square, triangle, paper, and masking tape, you will need the following:

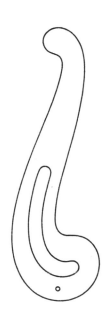

- A "light box" suitable for use with the T-square.
- Or transparent film or vellum for copying without a light box.
- Several technical pens of different point sizes, i.e., #1, #2, and #3 point pens.
- A symbol template (e.g. Sketch Mate Rapidesign, #19).
- Or a sheet of transfer symbols (e.g.Letraset key symbols, #2453)
- A French curve in a shape similar to the one shown at the left.
- Or pressure-sensitive, flexible black tape in $1/16$ or $1/32$ inch widths. Flex-a-Tape is one brand.
- An electric eraser and/or white paint, (e.g. Pro White opaque watercolor) and small brushes (e.g. Winsor Newton or Grumbcher red sable brushes, sizes 0, 00 or 000) for corrections.

Data should be plotted on graph paper in pencil, then copied in ink onto good paper. If you have a light box, use a plate finish bristol paper, one or two ply. Tape the bristol paper over the graph paper on the light box. When the light is turned on, it is easy to see the penciled graph lines for copying in ink.

Polyester drafting films, such as frosted Mylar, or a good quality, transparent vellum, such as Vidalon, can be used without a light box. Simply tape the film to the board over the penciled graph and copy in ink.

Axis Lines and Ticks

For axis lines and ticks, use the #1 and #0 pen respectively. Draw slow and steady lines against the T-square and triangle in the same way described on page 4 for tracings.

Design Symbols

For symbols, use the symbol template with a #2 pen. Practice with it first. You may find that if you fix tape to the solid parts of the template, it will lift it off the paper enough so that ink will not seep under the template. The best symbols to use are:

- Open and closed circles. ○ ● ○ ●
  Notice that the solid circles seem larger than the open circles. For equal emphasis, make the solid circle one size smaller. Above, the open circle is $5/32$ inch and the second closed circle is $1/8$ inch.
- Open and closed triangles. △ ▲ △ ▲
  Triangles in general look smaller than circles and in the second set, the open triangle is $3/16$ inch and the closed triangle is $5/32$ inch.
- Open and closed squares. □ ■ □ ■
  Squares look largest of all the symbols although the squares shown above are the same dimensions as the circles. In reduction, it may be difficult to distinguish between circles and squares. Triangles and circles are the easiest to distinguish in reduction.

The template on the left is a Sketch Mate Rapidesign, #19. Notice that this template contains hexagons. When used as graph symbols, hexagons look very similar to circles and in reduction, will not be distinguishable. (Hexagons are handy for chemical structures, however.)

Straight Lines

Straight lines connecting points are easily drawn with a ruler and a # 3 pen. If you stop short of the closed symbols, the symbol becomes better defined.

SPACE AROUND CLOSED SYMBOLS

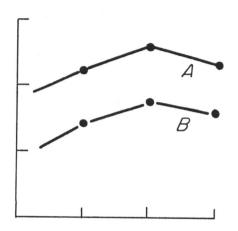

The #3 pen will give the heaviest line and when abutted to a symbol, tends to de-emphasize and possibly obscure it. This is shown in A. In B, the heavy line stops short of the symbols leaving space around them which serves as a white outline emphasizing the symbol.

Curved Lines

Curved lines done with the #3 pen against a **French curve** take practice. The French curve will generally only fit short segments of the curve, so that the curve will have to be repositioned often. It takes practice to draw the continuation of a line without being slightly offset from the original line.

To make a smooth curve quickly use **flexible tape**. Press the tape to the beginning of the curve, leaving some excess which may be trimmed exactly later on. Do not stretch the tape by pulling. Gently lay the tape along the curve pressing down with your finger when it is in the proper position. Trim the beginning and end of it with the cutting knife and a sharp blade. The tape must be patiently eased, and sometimes even cut, to accommodate sharp curves.

Label the Graph

Label the graph with any of the methods described above for tracings. The numbers and labels on the face of the graph, as for curves, should be the smallest size. The axes labels should be larger and are generally easier to read if they are upper and lower case. Make the title all upper case so that it will be the largest and most prominent label on the graph. (Or use upper and lower case in a larger font size). It is preferable not to use bold labels since they compete with the graphed data on the face of the graph. They also tend to thicken and blur in reduction.

Corrections

Corrections are almost always necessary and there are many methods for changing and improving.

- Small bumps or blobs on lines may be cleaned up with a small brush and white opaque paint . Use a magnifying glass for fine corrections.

- Irregular thicknesses of line may also be covered by applying transfer white lines such as Letraset # 223 arrows and lines in white. Cut the line to required dimensions and position it next to the straight line, covering the irregularities. Gently rub the line to transfer it .

- A symbol may be changed by applying white correction fluid (Lindsay's is one brand) and drawing another symbol over it after it has dried. Correction fluid, when dry, has a smoother surface than watercolor paint for accepting ink.

- A transfer label can be removed by covering it with masking tape and rubbing it down. When the tape is pulled off, the label will come with it.

- Lines, labels, symbols, and smudges may be removed by an electric eraser. With light pressure, it will remove ink from bristol, film, and vellum. To remove small areas of ink which are next to other areas you want to keep, use a metal eraser shield with the electric eraser.

Use a Photocopy Machine for Corrections and Changes

Many photocopying machines produce copies with excellent line quality which are suitable for print, slide, or poster. Many photographers prefer this kind of copy to originals with taped edges, white-outs, cut-and-pasted areas, and thin or grey lines. For slides, color may be added to photocopies using color film or markers. Photocopied transparencies may be used for overhead projectors or for figure overlays. Many photocopy machines permit enlargement or reduction and enlarged photocopies may be used for posters. Reduced photocopies are helpful for layouts, projections of reduction, insets, or making labeling changes.

A photocopying machine can be very helpful to:

- Eliminate unwanted material. Tape white paper over the unwanted area or cut it out and mount the desired area on white paper. Photocopy it using a normal setting.

- Add or exchange material. Cut and paste or tape additional or substitute material onto an existing figure. Photocopy the changed figure.

- Move material around and combine material by cutting and pasting.

- Enlarge or reduce labels by pasting or taping new labels over the old ones. This is illustrated on the next page.

LABELS TOO SMALL IN REDUCED GRAPH

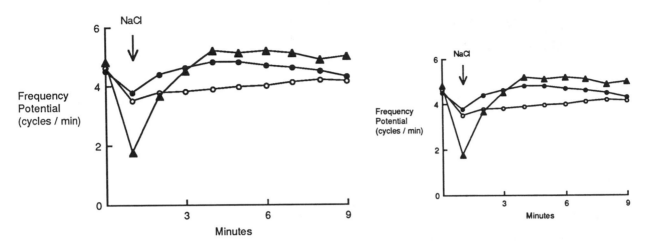

Although labels in the left-hand figure are readable, if this figure is reduced as on the right, the labels will be too small.

It is easier to cut and paste new labels than to redo them.

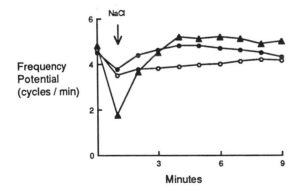

Here axes labels from an unreduced copy (above left) were cut out and pasted on top of a reduced figure (above right). This results in proportionally larger and more legible labels for a minimum of time and effort.

There are many ways to use the photocopy machine creatively to improve figures. For instance you can make a journal figure into a creditable slide by covering the caption and cutting and pasting or typing new labels and adding a title. (See *Chapter 10, Slides*).

With practice, you will develop skill and find shortcuts and new materials which will help you to do figures quickly and professionally. Use your imagination and visit stationery and art supply stores and study catalogs for new materials and tools that will serve your purpose.

Skill in the use of tools and materials for drawing give you independence and flexibility in getting figures done. Doing your own figures will also increase your knowledge and appreciation of good illustrations and make you more visually discriminating.

15

CONCLUSION

How often have I heard a researcher blame the audience for its failure to understand: "The information is obvious. If they don't understand it, that's their problem." In reality, the "problem" is the communicator's and it is serious.

Communicating information is not the same as doing research. Your data may be excellent and your analysis superb. You may be creative and imaginative at doing all the things necessary for fine research. No matter, these valuable traits will not automatically translate into clear communication.

It is ironic that today the best communicators communicate the most trivial information. Advertisers and ad agencies depend for their livelihood on selling an idea or product. They spend great amounts of time, energy, talent, and resources to do this.

ADVERTISEMENT

It's sort of like a tooth vitamin.

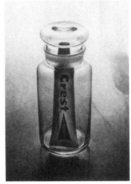

Crest similar to a vitamin?

Well, vitamins help keep your body strong. Crest does the same for your teeth. Vitamins help keep your body healthy. So does Crest for your teeth. Vitamins build up your body's resistance to disease. Crest builds up your teeth's resistance to cavities.

What makes Crest special is its fluoride, Fluoristan? And yet, most toothpastes don't have it. And that includes the leading toothpastes.

For example, take the five leading toothpastes. Only one contains the "tooth vitamin."

Of course, you know which one.

Ingenuity as well as thought, time, skill, and money went into this ad. The layout is simple and attractive; the analogy of toothpaste to vitamin is boldly and provocatively presented; the photograph reinforces the analogy; the text is concise. This figure attracts attention, then follows through with a clear, simple message.

In contrast, many scientists spend time, effort, and money to obscure and complicate serious, and sometimes, vital information.

SCIENTIFIC PRESENTATION

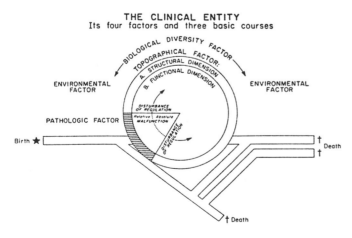

THE CLINICAL ENTITY
Its four factors and three basic courses

This figure has pretensions to erudition. Its simple message is that the course of disease has four factors and three outcomes. The wording obfuscates and the symbolism misleads.

Advertisers do not try to impress with learning. Advertisers do not try to confuse. Although some heap scorn on advertisers, we can learn a great deal from them about communicating.

You Should Learn To Communicate

In his book, *Information Anxiety*, Richard Saul Wurman talks about how we are "inundated with facts but starved for understanding". This sort of starvation is not only sad, but it is also dangerous for scientists. As the gap between the scientist and the public grows, public anxiety about scientific research increases and groups such as the animal rights enthusiasts gain strength.

This sort of starvation is also apparent in the failure of scientists to communicate clearly with other scientists. There is increasing specialization in scientific research and much greater complication of information. Unless a scientist is very clear and simple in the presentation of information, even other scientists may not understand.

This matters. It matters because the sharing of information among scientists is important for scientific progress. It matters because grants and jobs in science depend on communication. It matters because understanding of the world in which we live is important for our survival.

You Can Learn

We recognize a special skill involved in writing and speaking clearly and simply.

There is also a special skill in presenting visual information clearly and simply. Fortunately it is a skill which can be learned. It is a skill which the best of scientists have used and thought about, and one which is extremely useful for furtherance of science, career, and general knowledge. The drawings of Vesalius and his artists still speak to us, while his words do not. Pictures by Audubon and pictures of molecular structure are illuminating and astonishing.

Awareness

Awareness of standards, requirements, and means of making illustrations is the first step in learning visual communication.

- In order to utilize the services of an artist or photographer, you must be aware of what makes a good illustration.
- You must be aware of the limitations and assets of the media and materials that will be used.
- You must be aware of the illustrator's and photographer's informational needs and methods of working.

Awareness of your audience's background and level of knowledge will determine the kind of illustration which will communicate effectively.

Awareness of available choices are essential for good communication. This knowledge of existing choices should lead in turn to experimentation with new ways to express information visually.

Clear Purpose

If your own purpose is not clear, your figures will be confusing. Do not be afraid to be simple.

- Your general purpose should be to convey understanding through pictorial means.
- The purpose of individual figures must be clear and well thought out.
- Limit the amount of information in each figure.
- Emphasize what is important.

Time, Patience, and Practice

It takes time to learn about visual communication:

- Time to observe and think about your figures.
- Time to plan and organize your figures.
- Time to discuss your purpose and intentions with professionals in your field and in illustration.
- Time to do your own figures by computer or by hand.

Learning of any kind requires patience:

- Mistakes and errors are inevitable.
- Experience cannot be rushed, and in the meantime, the process, itself, can be enjoyable for you.
- Often the process of visualization and the making of visual choices can open your eyes and mind to further possibilities and challenges.

Practice is beneficial in many ways:

- The practice of focusing visually will sharpen your powers of analysis and observation.
- The practice of dealing with those who make figures for you will increase your knowledge of standards and methods of illustration.
- The practice of making your own figures will increase your efficiency and may open your eyes to other ways to illustrate.
- Practice can lead to experimentation, exploration and growth.

Pictures are a natural, easy, and interesting way of learning and should be used as one of the essential ways to increase understanding. Turgenev, the writer, acknowledged in *Fathers and Sons* that "A picture shows me at a glance what it takes dozens of pages of a book to expound".

BIBLIOGRAPHY

Alberts, B., Bray, D., Lewis, J., Raff, M., Roberts, K., Watson, J.D. Molecular biology of the cell. New York-London Garland, 1989.

Alder, H.L., Roessler, E.B. Introduction to probability and statistics. San Francisco Freeman, 1972.

Batschelet, E. Introduction to mathematics for life scientists. Volume 1. Berlin-Heidelberg-New York Springer-Verlag, 1971.

Baylor College of Medicine. Handbook for effective visuals. Medical illustration and audiovisual education, 1972.

Bojko, S. Diagrams, charts, graphs. Rhode Island School of Design. Graphis, 238. Zurich Graphis Press, 1985.

Cardamone, T. Chart and graph preparation skills. New York-Cincinnati Van Nostrand Teinhold, 1981.

Cleveland, W.S. The elements of graphing data. Monterey Wadsworth, 1985.

Croy, P. Graphic design and reproduction techniques. London-New York Focal, 1975.

Eastman Kodak. Communicating through poster sessions. No. P-319, 1978.
    -Effective lecture slides. S-22, 1981.
    -Legibility - artwork to screen. S-24, 1981
    -Planning and producing slide programs. S-30, 1981.

Edwards B. Drawing on the artist within. New York Simon and Schuster, 1986.

Herdeg, W. The artist in the service of science. Zurich Graphis, 1973.

Herrlinger, R. History of medical illustration. New York Medicina Rara, 1970.

Newman, J.R. The world of mathematics, Vol 1. New York Simon & Schuster, 1976.

Philadelphia Museum of Art. Ars medica. Art, medicine, and the human condition. Connecticut Meriden-Stinehour, 1985.

Simmonds, D. Charts and graphs. London MTP, 1980.

Stryer, L. Biochemistry. New York W.H. Freeman, 1988.

Trelease, S.F. How to write scientific and technical papers. Baltimore Williams and Wilkins, 1958.

Tufte, R. The visual display of quantitative information. New York Graphis, 1983.

Watson, J.D. Molecular biology of the gene. Menlo Park W.A. Benjamin, 1977.

Watson, J.D., Hopkins, N.H., Roberts, J.W., Steitz, J.A., Weiner, A.M. Molecular biology of the gene. Menlo Park Benjamin/Cummings, 1987.

Watson, S. Advertising: its role in modern marketing. New York Dunn-Holt-Reinholt-Winston, 1969.

Wurman, S.W. Information anxiety. New York Doubleday, 1989.

SOURCES OF ILLUSTRATIONS

PAGE   SOURCE

Chapter 1

4   Wayne B. Lanier, Ph.D.

Chapter 2

11- 14   Wayne B. Lanier, Ph.D.

Chapter 3

16 top   Tam K, Calonico LD, Nadel JA, McDonald DM. Globule leucocytes and mast cells in the rat trachea: their number, distribution and response to compound 48/80 and dexamethasone. Anatomy and Embryology 178(2): 95-190, 1988.

16 bottom   Wright JR, Clements JA. State of art: metabolism and turnover of lung surfactant. Am Rev Resp Dis, 135(1): 426-444, 1987.

17 top   Mary Helen Briscoe

17 bottom   Waldo Newberg, M.D.

18 top   Conhaim RL, Gropper MA, Staub N. Effect of lung inflation on alveolar-airway barrier protein permeability in dog lung. J Appl Physiol 55(4): 1249-1256, 1983.

18 bottom   Joan Wikman-Coffelt. Biochemical regulation of myocardial hypertrophy. Handbook of Hypertension, Vol 7: Pathophysiology of Hypertension-Cardiovascular Aspects, A. Zanchetti and R.C. Tarazi, editors, 1986.

19 top   Davis B, Nadel JA. New methods to investigate control of mucus secretion and ion transport in airways. Environ. Health Perspective 35: 121-130, 1980.

19 bottom   Jay A. Nadel, M.D.

20   Waldo Newberg, M.D.

Chapter 4

25	Mary Helen Briscoe. Tracings courtesy of William H. Tooley, M.D. and Mureen Schleuter.
26	Mary Helen Briscoe
27	Wolfe CH, Moseley ME, Wikstrom MG, et al. Assessment of myocardial salvage after ischemia and reperfusion using magnetic resonance imaging and spectroscopy. Circulation 1989, in press. (Oct. '89). By permission of the American Heart Association, Inc.
29	Michael A. Heymann, M.D.
30-34	Mary Helen Briscoe
35 top	Michael A. Heymann, M.D.
35 bottom	Mary Helen Briscoe. Photomicrographs courtesy of Robert L. Hamilton, Jr., Ph.D. and John P. Kane M.D., Ph.D.
36 top	Mary Helen Briscoe. Photomicrographs courtesy of Robert L. Hamilton, Jr., Ph.D. and John P. Kane M.D., Ph.D.
36 bottom	Mary Helen Briscoe
37-39	G. Chi Chen, Ph.D, David Hardman
40-41	Mary Helen Briscoe. Echocardiogram courtesy of Nelson B. Schiller, M.D.

Chapter 5

44	Wayne B. Lanier, Ph.D.
45 top	Mary Helen Briscoe. Adapted from the following figure.
45 bottom	Henry Edmunds, M.D.
46	Norman C. Staub, M.D. To be published. Modern Physiology of Respiration. Chicago Year Book Medical Publishers, Inc., 1989.
49	Bland RD, McMillan DD, Bressack MA. Decreased pulmonary transvascular fluid filtration in awake newborn lambs after intravenous furosemide. Reproduced from the Journal of Clinical Investigation, 1978, 62 (3): 601-609, by copyright permission of the American Society for Clinical Investigation.
50, 51, 53	Mary Helen Briscoe. Adapted from the preceding figure.
54	Mary Helen Briscoe. Created from data contained in the table on page 49.

55	Landolt CC, Matthay MA, Albertine KH, Roos PH, Wiener-Kronish JP, Staub NC. Overperfusion, hypoxia and increased pressure cause only hydrostatic pulmonary edema in anesthetized sheep. Circ Res 52: 335-341, 1983, by permission of the American Heart Association, Inc.

Chapter 6

58	Jori Mandelman
59-62 top	Mary Helen Briscoe. Adapted from the preceding figure.
62 bottom	Jori Mandelman
63	Mary Helen Briscoe. Adapted from the preceding figure.
65 top	Mary Helen Briscoe
65 bottom	Jori Mandelman
66	Mary Helen Briscoe. Adapted from the preceding figure.
67 left	J. Mandelman
67 right	Mary Helen Briscoe. Adapted from the figure to the left.
68	Jori Mandelman
69 top	Chuen -Shang C. Wu, Ph.D., Jen Tsi Yang, Ph.D.
69 bottom	Adapted from Richardson JS. Anatomy and taxonomy of protein structure. Academic Press. Advances in protein chemistry Vol. 34: 168-364, 1981. For Chuen-Shang C. Wu and Jen Tsi Yang.
70-71	Mary Helen Briscoe

Chapter 7

76	Mary Helen Briscoe
77	Mary Helen Briscoe. Adapted from data from Terjung RJ, Baldwin KM, Winder WW, Holloszy JO. Glycogen repletion in different types of muscle and in liver after exhausting exercise. Am J Physiol 226, 6, 1974.
78 top	Mary Helen Briscoe. From Terjung, et al., op. cit.
78 bottom	Mary Helen Briscoe
79 top, middle	Mary Helen Briscoe
79 bottom	Mary Helen Briscoe. From Terjung, et al., op. cit., pg. 77.
80 top	Mary Helen Briscoe. From Terjung, et al., op. cit.
80 bottom	Mary Helen Briscoe
81 top	Mary Helen Briscoe

81 bottom   Mary Helen Briscoe. From Terjung, et al., op. cit., pg. 77.

82   Mary Helen Briscoe

Chapter 8

83-85   Mary Helen Briscoe. From Terjung, et al., op. cit., pg 77.

86   Mary Helen Briscoe

87   Mary Helen Briscoe. From Terjung, et al., op. cit., pg. 77.

88   Mary Helen Briscoe

89   Mary Helen Briscoe. From Terjung, et al., op. cit., pg. 77.

90 top   Mary Helen Briscoe

90 bottom   Mary Helen Briscoe. From Terjung, et al., op. cit., pg. 77.

91 top   Mary Helen Briscoe. From Terjung, et al., op. cit.

91 bottom   Mary Helen Briscoe

92   Mary Helen Briscoe

93-103   Mary Helen Briscoe. From Terjung, et al., op. cit., pg. 77.

104-106   Mary Helen Briscoe

107   Mary Helen Briscoe. From Terjung, et al., op. cit., pg. 77.

Chapter 9

111-117   Mary Helen Briscoe

118-119   Mary Helen Briscoe. From Terjung, et al., op. cit., pg. 77.

Chapter 10

123-124   Mary Helen Briscoe. Modified from *A Guide to illustrations for medical and scientific research*. Regents, University of California, 1986.

125-126   Mary Helen Briscoe

127-129   Mary Helen Briscoe. From Terjung, et al., op. cit., pg. 77.

132   Hotkins AL, Koprowski H. How the immune response to a virus can cause disease. Sci Am 228(1): 24. 1973.

Chapter 11

136-137   Mary Helen Briscoe

139   From meeting instructions to authors.

140   Mary Helen Briscoe

142-144   Mary Helen Briscoe

145   Baker DG and Don H. Catecholamines abolish vagal but not acetylcholine tone in the intact cat trachea. J Appl Physiol 63(6): 2490-2498. 1987

Chapter 12

156   Mary Helen Briscoe

158-159   Mary Helen Briscoe

163-164   Mary Helen Briscoe from Wayne B. Lanier, Ph.D.

165   Mary Helen Briscoe

166-167   Morales M. Science as a way of knowing. American Zoologist, in press 1989.

169-170   Mary Helen Briscoe

Chapter 13

175   Mary Helen Briscoe

177-180   Mary Helen Briscoe

182   Chuen-Shang C. Wu, Ph.D and Jen Tsi Yang, Ph.D.

183-185   Mary Helen Briscoe

188   Mary Helen Briscoe

Chapter 14

192 top   Courtesy of the Proctor & Gamble Company.

192 bottom   Otto E. Guttentag, M.D. The attending physician as a central figure. Changing Values in Medicine. Edited by E.J. Cassell and M. Siegler. Frederick, Maryland, University Publishers of America. 1979.

INDEX